The Baby Bible [2 in 1]

Learn how to Treat ADHD, Overcome Conflicts and Grow Happy Children in 2021

By

Laura Candice

and is universal as so. The presentation of the information is without contract or any type of guarantee assurance.

The trademarks that are used are without any consent, and the publication of the trademark is without permission or backing by the trademark owner. All trademarks and brands within this book are for clarifying purposes only and are the owned by the owners themselves, not affiliated with this document.

Author: Laura Candice

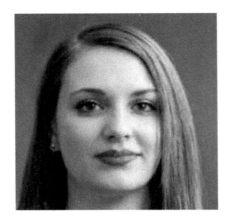

Laura Candice is an experience mom of three real kids who live a happy life outside Seattle with her husband. She is also the creator of 7+ incredible works that led her to become a real guru in the field of education between parents and children. Laura has a degree in elementary education, eight years of teaching experience and a pure passion for early childhood learning. Susie's advices have inspired hundreds of thousands of parents through her real, hands-on approach to real parenting.

All her view of life can be summarized in her current motto: "Parents can only give good advice or put it on the right path, but the final formation of a person's character lies in his own hands."

Table of Contents

Anger Management For Kids [with Exercises]

Potty Training in 3 Days

Anger Management For Kids [with Exercises]

19+ Brain-Improving Activities to Reduce Meltdowns, Increase Positive Behaviors and Manage Emotions

By

Laura Candice

Table of Contents

INTRODUCTION

Do you often find yourself in trouble because of anger? Do you react to situations and later regret how you behaved? Does your anger cause problems with other people? Are you tired of letting anger control you? If you answered yes to any of these questions, *Anger Management for Kids* is for you.

First and foremost, it is important to understand that anger is a natural human emotion, but people handle it differently. Some hold in their anger and let it build, some lash out with hurtful words, some resort to fighting, and some just explode. No matter how you handle it, you are reading this book because you or someone who cares about you thinks you have a problem with anger.

You are not alone. Anger affects millions of teens, who often find themselves lonely and depressed. They may feel like their relationships are less meaningful or as though they just don't care anymore.

The activities in this workbook will help you notice things that make you angry, handle frustrating situations without getting angry, and effectively communicate your feelings. Most of all, these activities can help you learn to change how you respond to anger. Change is not easy, but with the right frame of mind and set of skills, you can do it. So, let's get started!
Wishing you success.

Exercise 1 your anger profile

---

for you to know

While each person's experience with anger is different, it's important to recognize your own personal profile so you can learn to head off anger before it gets the best of you. Assessing your anger will help you become moreaware of how much it drives your behavior.

Terrence was having a really bad day. Mr. Williams, Terrence's English teacher, noticed that he seemed angry about something. "Oh no," thought Mr. Williams, "Terrence is in one of his moods. He's so smart and talented, but his anger is really hurting him. He's going to get into trouble if he doesn't turn it around."

After class, Mr. Williams called Terrence over and said, "You take everything so seriously, Terrence. Your anger is beginning to get in the way of your schoolwork, and I'm really worried about you. You've been suspended three times this year and you're constantly in the principal's office. Let me help you. What do you say?"

Terrence knew that Mr. Williams was right. So, he nodded his head and said, "Yeah, okay...."

"Great," Mr. Williams said. "We'll begin by taking a good look at your anger. Once we see what effect it has on you, we can start to come up with a plan to help you manage it."

For you to do

This Exercise will help you gauge how much of a problem your angeris and begin to understand how it affects your life.

Read each statement and check either "Yes" or "No."

People have often commented on my anger.   ☐ Yes   ☐ No

My anger gets me into trouble.   ☐ Yes   ☐ No

I have occasionally become so angry that later I could not remember what I did.   ☐ Yes   ☐ No

Other members of my family have anger problems.   ☐ Yes   ☐ No

I have hit or harmed someone else when I was angry.   ☐ Yes   ☐ No

I often feel that I am the victim.   ☐ Yes   ☐ No

I often feel that no one understands me.   ☐ Yes   ☐ No

For each of these statements, circle the number that best describes you.

I have trouble controlling my anger.

1	2	3	4	5
strongly disagree	disagree	neutral	agree	strongly agree

On average, I get really angry ...

1	2	3	4	5
once a month	every two weeks	once a week	every few days	every day

When I get angry, I am most likely to ...

1	2	3	4	5
run away from the situation	cry	scream	hit something	destroy something

The more frequently you checked "Yes" and the higher you rated yourself on these scales, the more anger is driving your life. By committing to doing the activities in this book, you will learn skills that will help you get a grip on youranger.

… and more to do!

Has your anger ever hurt you emotionally or physically? Tell how.

_____

_____

_____

Do you ever blame others for your anger? Tell how (for example, by makingaccusations or denying that you did something).

_____

_____

_____

When you are angry, do you frequently say or do things that you later regret?

Describe a time when this happened.

_____

_____

_____

What do you do to calm down when you're angry? Does it work?

_____

_____

_____

If you could change one thing about yourself, what would it be?

_____

_____

_____

Exercise 2 making a game plan

---

for you to know

Making a game plan is a great way to tackle changing things about yourself that are causing you problems. When you make something a priority, you'll be more motivated to get it done. And, the more motivated you are, the harder you'll work to change.

There are thirty-six more activities in this workbook. If you try to do an Exercise a day, you may be rushing through the workbook and not getting the full benefit.If you do two or three a week, you will have time to think about what you are learning and apply it to your life.

Give yourself time to do each Exercise and to practice using some of the skills you are learning before taking on the next one. It's important to do all of the activities in the order they appear. The skills become more complex as you go along, and each Exercise builds on the ones that precede it.

Here are some important things to remember as you develop your plan:

- Schedule a time to work on your activities and treat the time like anassignment. You'll be more likely to stick to your plan that way.

- Practice the skills you are learning. The more something is part of youreveryday life, the more likely you are to change.

- Don't fly through the activities. Go slowly and reflect on what you havelearned.

- Focus on what you've already accomplished as opposed to what you stillhave left to do. The remaining job will then seem more manageable.

for you to do

Write out a schedule for working on the activities. If something comes up and you have to change your plan, that's okay. In fact, you may want to do this Exercise in pencil so you can go back and make changes.

Anger Workbook Schedule		
Date to Begin	Activity	Date Completed
	3. Setting Goals and Creating Action Plans	
	4. Rewarding Yourself	
	5. Keeping an Anger Log	
	6. Recognizing Your Anger Buttons	
	7. Understanding Family Patterns	
	8. Your Body's Response to Anger	
	9. Fight or Flight	
	10. Masking Your Emotions	
	11. The Media and Anger	
	12. Using Anger for Positive Results	
	13. Chilling Out	
	14. Writing	
	15. Laughing at Anger	
	16. Taking a Mental Vacation	
	17. Releasing Anger Symbolically	
	18. Relaxation Techniques	

Date to Begin	Activity	Date Completed
	19. Handling Anger Constructively	
	20. Anger Contract	
	21. Taking Responsibility for Your Own Actions	
	22. Keeping Perspective	
	23. Getting the Facts	
	24. Stages of Anger	
	25. Perception	
	26. Weighing the Options	
	27. The ABC Model of Anger	
	28. Coping with Conflict	
	29. Using I-Messages	
	30. Good Listening	
	31. Complimenting Others	
	32. Body Language	
	33. Communicating Clearly	
	34. Being Assertive	
	35. Steps Toward Change	
	36. Seeing How Far You Have Come	
	37. Anger Certificate	

… and more to do!

You can increase your chances of sticking to your plan by following these tips:

- Work on the activities at the same time daily, such as right after school.

- Commit to working on the activities for a set amount of time each day, perhaps fifteen minutes.

- Tell a trusted friend that you're working on the activities so that you have someone supporting you as you make progress.

What other ways can you think of to increase your chances of sticking to yourplan?

_____

_____

_____

What goals have you had in the past that required you to make a game plan?

_____

_____

_____

Do you think having a plan helped you achieve those goals? Tell why or whynot.

_____

_____

_____

Do you have any other goals that might benefit from a plan? If so, what arethey?

_____

_____

_____

setting goals and creating action plans

---

for you to know

There are two types of goals: short-term and long-term. Short-term goals are ones you will achieve in the near future, such as within a day or a week. Long-term goals are ones you will achieve in a longer period of time, such as a month or a year. The steps you take to achieve your goals make up your action plan.

Antonio was constantly in trouble. He was failing two courses and he was always fighting with his parents. If he didn't like how other kids looked at him, he was in their faces in a heartbeat: "What are you looking at, punks!" Shoving, pushing, talking back, and slamming things around were his ways of dealing with life.

One day, Antonio realized that it was time for a change. The person he had become on the outside wasn't his real self. He felt like he was in a tug-of-war with his anger — and his anger was winning. He went to see his school counselor, Ms. Lee, who offered to help him.

"The first step," said Ms. Lee, "is to develop some goals. Think of a mountain climber who starts at the foot of a mountain. His long-term goal is to reach the summit before nightfall. He breaks up the climb into smaller segments so that it doesn't seem so overwhelming; those segments are his short-term goals. He also has an action plan, which is his strategy for reaching each goal. You can take the same approach to getting your anger under control."

Long-Term Goal: I will control my anger.

Action Plan:

1. I will learn to talk about what bothers me rather than getting angry.

2. I will learn to compromise.

3. I will learn to focus on the positive side of situations.

Short-Term Goal: I will fight less often in the next month.

Action Plan:

1. I will not provoke, name-call, push, or hit anyone.

2. I will ask for help when I feel frustrated.

3. I will take ten deep breaths when I find myself wanting to yell at my parents.

Working with Ms. Lee, Antonio came up with these goals and actions plans.With his goals and plan in place, Antonio was on his way to change.

for you to do

Setting goals for yourself is an important step toward change. In thespace that follows, write down two anger goals for yourself: one long-term and one short-term. Then add your action plans, which are the steps you will take to reach each goal.

My Anger Goals and Action Plans Long-Term Goal:

_____

_____

Action Plan: _____

_____

_____

_____

Short-Term Goal: _____

_____

Action Plan: _____

_____

_____

_____

... and more to do!

What other areas of your life would benefit from your setting goals and creating an action plan? Some possibilities include school, work, and relationships.

_____

_____

_____

Choose one of these areas, and set a long-term goal and a short-term goal. Then create an action plan for these goals.

Long-Term Goal: _____

_____

Action Plan: _____

_____

_____

_____

Short-Term Goal: _____

_____

Action Plan: _____

_____

_____

_____

Exercise 4 rewarding yourself

---

for you to know

It's a good idea to reward yourself when you accomplish one of your anger-management goals. Why? The answer is simple: It makes you feel good! And that's not the only reason. Rewards are motivating, and the more motivation you have to do something, the harder you'll try.

Learning to manage your anger isn't going to be easy, but rewards can help youreach your goals. A reward provides you with motivation to do something that might otherwise be hard for you. For example, if you're trying to stop yelling atyour mom, your reward might be that you get to blog on the computer if you make it through dinner without yelling. The goal is not to yell, and the reward isblogging on the computer.

Here are some other rewards you might choose:

- seeing a movie

- downloading new musicshopping

- going to a concert

- eating out at your favorite restauranthanging out with friends

    skateboarding

- riding your bikeshooting hoops

for you to do

Next to each treasure chest, write down what you would like to reward yourself with and the date you will try to earn the reward by. When you have reached a goal, write down what you achieved. Tryto earn all your rewards!

I will work to achieve this reward: _____

I plan to earn this reward by this date: _____

To earn this reward, I _____

_____

I will work to achieve this reward: _____

I plan to earn this reward by this date: _____

To earn this reward, I _____

_____

I will work to achieve this reward: _____

I plan to earn this reward by this date: _____

To earn this reward, I _____

_____

I will work to achieve this reward: _____

I plan to earn this reward by this date: _____

To earn this reward, I _____

_____

... and more to do!

Look back at the goals you set in Exercise 3 and share them with a friend or family member whom you trust. Ask this person to notice when you meet one of your goals and to remind you to give yourself a reward. Keep a record of all the goals you've achieved and rewards you've received. If you become discouraged, you can look back at this Exercise and see how far you've come!

I Did It!		
Goal I Reached	Reward I Received	Date I Received It

Exercise 5 keeping an anger log

Michelle had been waiting all week for Alicia to come over for a sleepover. They had big plans for Saturday night, and Michelle was literally counting down the minutes. Saturday morning around ten, Alicia texted her: "no good 4 2nite. have 2 do it another time." "Are you for real?" Michelle thought.

This wasn't the first time Alicia had stood Michelle up. She felt like she couldn't count on Alicia for anything. The more she thought about it, the angrier she became. Before she knew it, Michelle grabbed a shoe and threw it at the wall — hard. It landed on her desk and knocked over some pictures, which fell and broke. Her parents heard the commotion and ran to her room, only to find a mess. The result? Michelle was grounded for two weeks.

Later that afternoon, when Michelle had calmed down, her mom said to her, "Honey, you seem to get angry at Alicia so often, and the results are never good. It might help if you could see the patterns. That way, you could start to think about more helpful ways to react."

Keeping a log can help you see patterns in your anger. This sample entry shows you how Michelle might have recorded what happened with Alicia.

Anger Log	
Date and Time:	October 3, 10 a.m.
What Happened:	Alicia texted last minute and can't stay over.
What I Was Thinking:	She always makes excuses. I am sick of being her friend.
What I Was Feeling:	Furious, disappointed, and hurt
What I Did:	Threw a shoe at my desk
What My Consequences Were:	Trouble with parents. Broke some of my favorite pictures. Grounded for two weeks.
How I Handled It:	Not well. I am going to be a hermit for the next few weeks. Not to mention I have a mess to clean up.
What I Could Have Done Instead:	Told Alicia that I was angry about her constant excuses, then called another friend to come over or asked my sister if she was up for a movie.

for you to do

Before you start, make several photocopies of this blank log. For as long as you are working on the activities in this book, keep your anger log.

Anger Log	
Date and Time:	
What Happened:	
What I Was Thinking:	
What I Was Feeling:	
What I Did:	
What My Consequences Were:	
How I Handled It:	
What I Could Have Done Instead:	

… and more to do!

Once you've made a few entries in your log, see if you notice a pattern of when you get angry.

Is there any particular time of the day when this occurs (for example, in the evening when you are tired or trying to do homework, or in the morning when you first wake up)?

_____

_____

_____

Do you seem to get angry in certain situations or with particular people?

_____

_____

_____

Are there specific areas you think you can work on?

_____

_____

_____

After a few weeks, review your log. Have you seen an improvement in the wayyou handle your anger? If so, tell what has changed.

_____

_____

_____

Exercise 6 recognizing your anger buttons

---

for you to know

We all have buttons that when pushed lead to anger. Some people call these buttons "pet peeves" or "triggers." No matter what you call them, it's important that you identify the things that bug you and head them off before your anger builds.

Tabitha came up to Leigha in the hall and accused her of taking Jessica's textbook from her locker. Leigha hadn't even gone to Jessica's locker! She tried to explain, but Tabitha interrupted and said, "Josh told us he saw you in Jessica's locker this morning, and now her history book is missing. Her homework was inside that book. Just give it back so she doesn't get a bad grade."

Leigha's fists clenched, and she raised her voice. "Tabitha, for the last time, I don't have Jessica's stuff!" But Tabitha would not back down. She got right in Leigha's face and called her a liar. That did it! Being accused of lying always set Leigha off. She threw down her books and knocked Tabitha's stuff out of her hands. "You did not just call me a liar!"

Just like Leigha, we all have things that push our buttons. Here are some examples of things others do that may push your buttons:

- Nag you

- Tell others something you told them in confidenceTry to boss you around

- Accuse you of something you didn't do
- Invade your space

- Accuse you of saying something you didn't sayMake repetitive noises

- Borrow something of yours without permissionBorrow something of yours and ruin it

- Write nasty things about youGo through your things

for you to do

In the column headed "Button," write down things that are very likely to set off your anger. In the next column, write down one thingyou can do to release that button when you realize it is being pushed. For example, if being nagged is one of your buttons, you may be able to release it by removing yourself from the situation. Finally, rank your buttons from most annoying to least annoying.

Button	Release	Rank

How can knowing what your buttons are help you with anger?

_____

_____

_____

... and more to do!

On a separate sheet of paper, list your button releases and then make several copies of your list. Put them in places that are readilyaccessible — for example, your wallet, your backpack, and your nightstand. Review the list often so that the next time you find one of your buttons is being pushed, you can head off an angersituation by recalling your release.

Exercise 7 Understanding family patterns

for you to know

You've probably spent a lot of time around your family, especially when you were little, so naturally you've picked up some of your habits and behaviors from them. Exploring how members of your family interact can help you understand your own response to anger.

Gabrielle's dad had given her a list of chores to do before she could go to the mall with her friends. The more she thought about all the things she had to do, the more upset she got. "Clean this, do that," she muttered. "Do it yourself, Dad!"

Her father heard her and yelled, "If I hear one more smart word out of your mouth, you won't go anywhere! Do I make myself clear?"

"Perfectly!" said Gabrielle, rolling her eyes. She stomped off. She picked up her clothes from the floor and tossed them into the laundry room, kicking the door on her way out. Next, she started to unload the dishwasher. She threw the silverware into the drawer and banged pots around as she put them away.

Her father marched into the kitchen and slammed his hand on the counter. "Listen here, young lady, stop banging stuff around!"

Just then Gabrielle's mother walked into the room. "What on earth is going on here? All I hear is screaming and slamming. You two are like peas in a pod. Gabrielle, you get that temper from your dad's side. They all throw temper tantrums when they don't get their way. Both of you, settle down and get away from each other for a while. Gabrielle, you know the rule: no privileges unless you do your chores. If you're not done in an hour, then you can't go to the mall."

"Okay," Gabrielle sighed. She knew that her mom meant what she said.

for you to do

At the bottom of this tree, write your name. Then add the names of your family members. In the space provided, indicate how they handle anger, such as:

- blows up

- walks away from the situationyells

- throws things goes for a jog holds anger insidesays mean things

- takes some time alone to calm down

- On or near the tree, add the names of other family members — aunts, uncles,cousins, or siblings, for example — whom you have been told you are like.

Circle the name of the person you most resemble in your response to anger. Inthe space provided, indicate how your parents and grandparents handle anger.

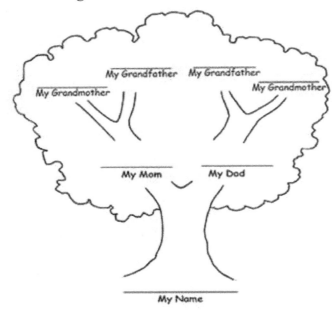

… and more to do!

Did you notice a pattern in how your relatives handle anger? If so, explain.

_____

_____

_____

What was one thing that stood out about how your family members deal withtheir anger?

_____

_____

_____

Choose one family member who manages anger well. Tell what you can do to tryto be more like that person.

_____

_____

_____

Exercise 8
your body's response to anger

---

for you to know

Anger causes stress, which can lead to physical reactions that include high blood pressure, headaches, stomachaches,and heart problems, among others. Not everyone reacts thesame way, and learning how anger affects your body will help you recognize when you are becoming angry.

Look at some of the physical ways anger manifests itself. When you get angry,you might experience some of these things:

- cry

- feel your face get hotgrind your teeth

- roll your eyes breathe heavily

- notice that your heart is racingbreak out in a rash

- feel short of breathget a headache

- get a stomachache
- sweat

- have nervous twitches feel your muscles tightenfeel dizzy

- feel nauseated

Knowing your physical response to anger can help you become aware of whenyou need to cool it. These tips can help when you reach that point:

- Take five deep breaths, concentrating on exhaling.

- Excuse yourself from the situation and go for a walk or go to a quiet space.

- If you can't get away from the situation, you can tell yourself to calm down and imagine a relaxing place (perhaps your bedroom, the beach, or your grandmother's house). As you bring this place to mind, focus on letting the anger drain from your body like water from a bathtub.

for you to do

In the outline below, draw in all the parts of your body that are affected when you feel angry. For example, if you cry when you get angry, you might draw eyes with tears. If your muscles get tight, you might draw flexed biceps.

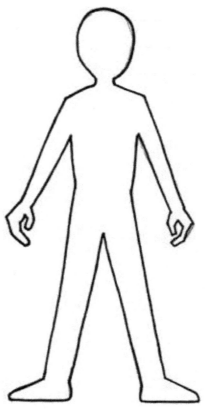

... and more to do!

How does your body respond to anger?

_____

_____

_____

What part of your body is most affected by anger?

_____

_____

_____

In addition to the earlier suggestions, what else can you do to cool down whenyou feel your body responding to anger?

_____

_____

_____

_____

Exercise 9 fight or flight

---

for you to know

Each time you sense danger, your body automatically tries to protect you. Adrenaline, a chemical that gives you a quick rush of energy, is released into your bloodstream. Your pupils dilate, your heart rate accelerates, your blood pressure rises, and your breathing speeds up. You become alert and highly sensitive to your surroundings. This combination of reactions is called the fight-or-flight response. How you react to this response can improve situations or make them worse.

Lisa got home from school and went straight to the computer. To her surprise, when she opened Facebook, there was a nasty message from a girl in her math class. "How dare she slam me like that! Who does she think she is?" Lisa thought.

As Lisa continued to read, she wondered, "How many people have seen this? She's ruined my life!" And the more she read, the angrier she became. Her face started to get hot, and her shoulder muscles began to tense. All she could think was: "I'll get her back!"

Lisa was faced with a choice: fight or flight. What do you think she chose? If you guessed fight, you're right. Instead of withdrawing, she reacted by wanting to get back at the other girl.

When you feel your body going into this mode, you can react positively or negatively. Positive reactions can improve the situation, while negative ones only make things worse.

for you to do

Read this situation; put a "P" next to positive reactions and an "N" next to negative reactions.

William had prepared all week for his in-class presentation. When he got up to speak, he noticed his classmates were whispering. Some kids were looking at him and snickering. He tried to concentrate on his presentation, but his mind went blank. When the teacher prompted him to start, he broke into a cold sweat and stared out across the room. All he could think was: "These kids are ruining it for me!" What is William going to do?

_____Block the class out mentally and try to pretend that they don't exist.

_____Stop and ask to speak with the teacher in private.

_____Run out of the room.

_____Say something like, "Hey, guys, give me a break."

_____Yell at the class for messing up his presentation.

_____Throw his materials across the room while screaming, "I've had it!"

Next, read these situations and come up with your own ideas for positive reactions.

Bianca had tried out for the lead in the school play. She really thought she deserved the part, and today the drama coach was posting the cast list. At lunchtime, Bianca joined the crowd of kids at the bulletin board. She read down the list, and her face turned bright red when she saw that Arielle had gotten the lead. And what was worse, Bianca was going to be in the chorus. She wouldn't even have any lines! Just then, Arielle walked up and several of the kids congratulated her. Bianca felt like stomping off. What could she do?

_____

_____

_____

Molly was always borrowing Kim's iPod. One Friday afternoon, Kim asked Molly to return it. "Uh, I don't have it. I let Ian borrow it," Molly replied. Kim couldn't believe her ears. Molly had no right to lend something that didn't even belong to her! Kim was furious with Molly, but she'd deal with that later. First she needed to find Ian and get her iPod back. As Kim approached Ian, she noticed he was holding an iPod — and it looked broken! Her heart started to pound. What could she do?

_____

_____

_____

… and more to do!

Think of a time when your body went into fight-or-flight mode. Describe the situation.

_____

_____

_____

How did your body react?

_____

_____

_____

Tell how you handled the situation and whether you think your response waspositive or negative.

_____

_____

_____

Can you think of other positive reactions you might have had?

_____

_____

_____

Exercise 10 masking your emotions

for you to know

Sometimes it's easier to get mad than to admit that your feelings are hurt or that you're really scared. But masking other emotions with anger is not a positive way to cope with a situation, and it can actually be harmful. Until you deal with your underlying feelings, your anger may continue to grow.

Jake could tell something was up at home. His parents had been arguing constantly. His dad often left and didn't come home until one or two in the morning. His mom cried a lot, and Jake had seen her sitting in the kitchen with a checkbook and calculator, looking worried. Once he overheard them discussing whom he would live with if they separated.

Jake felt anxious about the future and hurt that his parents hadn't told him what was happening. He also felt a bit guilty because he wondered if he was the cause of their arguments.

Finally, one Saturday at breakfast, his parents told him that they would be getting a divorce. Jake immediately felt his stomach knot and his face turn red. He shouted, "That's the worst! I don't even want to talk about it!" He jumped up and stormed away from the table.

His mom called him back. She looked at him closely and said, "Jake, you look so angry, but I know you must have other feelings about this divorce. Let's talk about them." When Jake was able to express the feelings that lay under his anger, he began to feel calmer.

for you to do

This list represents some feelings you may have masked with anger. Circle any that apply to you, and use the blank lines to add others.

hurt	depression	fear
greed	stress	shame
anxiety	frustration	_____
loneliness	jealousy	_____

Tell about a specific time when you masked your feelings with anger.

_____

_____

_____

How would expressing your actual feelings have helped?

_____

_____

_____

... and more to do!

Choose another situation that made you angry and then think about what other emotions might have been at the root of your anger. In the mask below, write down those feelings. If you prefer, you can use the space to create a collage of pictures or words from old magazines or newspapers. When you have finished, look at your mask and think about how you let each of those feelings get replaced by anger.

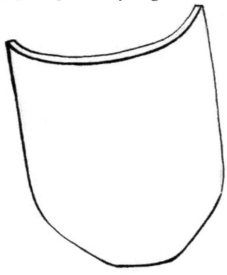

Exercise 11
the media and anger

---

for you to know

The more that people see violence in the media, the more likely they are to act out aggressively. If you reduce your exposure to violent TV shows and video games, you will find it easier to manage your anger.

Did you know that the level of violent behavior in Saturday morning cartoons is higher than in prime-time television? Children's TV shows depict even more violence than shows for adults do, so from the time you were a young child to today, it's likely that you've watched a lot of anger and aggression on TV shows. And TV is not the only source of exposure to violence. Movies, music videos, video games, newspapers, magazines, and the Internet all contribute to the amount of violence you see.

The fast-paced, intense action may get you involved and hold your attention, but it's actually bad for you. Studies have shown that watching lots of violent shows or playing violent games can cause people to react aggressively.

for you to do For one week, keep a record of how often you are exposed to violence in the media. In the bottom row, add up the incidents of violence. You may be surprised at how much anger and aggression you're seeing!

	Television	Movies	Music Videos	Video Games	Newspapers and Magazines	The Internet
Monday						
Tuesday						
Wednesday						
Thursday						
Friday						
Saturday						
Sunday						
Total						

Which type of media exposed you to the most violence?_____

Adding all columns, how much media violence were you exposed to over theweek?

_____

What are your thoughts about the amount of media violence you see?

_____

_____

_____

... and more to do!

Are there certain TV shows or video games you could cut out ofyour life? Write their titles here.

_____

_____

_____

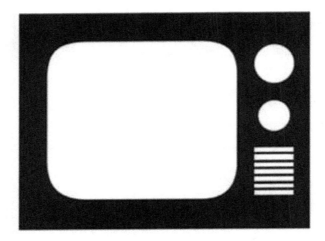

Make a pledge to reduce the level of media violence you are exposed to.
Write ithere: _____

_____

_____

Exercise 12
using anger for positive results

---

for you to know

Even though anger has a bad rap, it can be a very useful emotion. Expressing your anger is one way to stand up for your rights and the rights of others. It can help you promote change when you think something is unfair. For example, if Martin Luther King Jr. had not gotten angry, there would be a lot more injustice in this world.

Nathan was on his way home when he saw a boy pushing around a smaller boy. He watched for a minute as the bully kept shoving the other kid. The poor kid didn't have a chance; each time he got up, the bully would shove him again, and he would stumble and fall to the ground.

"That's not right," Nathan thought. "That guy is twice his size. He's going to hurt that kid." He walked toward the bully and called, "Hey, stop! Why don't you leave him alone?"

The bully turned and looked at Nathan. "Why don't you mind your own business?" he responded.

Nathan, who was much taller than the bully, grinned and said, "This is my business."

The bully gave another glance at Nathan. Then he turned back to the kid and said, "You're not worth my time." He headed off.

Nathan went over to the kid. "Are you all right?"

"Yeah," said the kid. "That guy's a real jerk; he pushes everyone around. Thanks for your help."

The next week, Nathan was still really bothered by what had happened, so he met with the principal at his school. He suggested that the students develop a club to teach kids how to stand up against bullies and how to get help from adults. The principal was very excited about Nathan's idea and said, "Nathan, your anger about seeing another student get pushed around will lead to a wonderful program to help others avoid that experience!"

Next time you find yourself getting angry, take your anger and turn it to good. Ask yourself these questions:

- What is within my control?

- How can I be an agent for change?

- What can I do to fix the problem rather than just acting out in anger?

Remember, anger itself is not necessarily a problem. It's how you choose to handle it.

for you to do

Think of a time when you turned your anger into something positive, perhaps by standing up for someone in a difficult situation, or protesting against something you thought was unfair.

Describe the situation.

_____

_____

_____

Tell how you handled the situation.

_____

_____

_____

Are you satisfied with how you reacted? If not, what could you have donedifferently?

_____

_____

_____

... and more to do!

When people use their anger to stick up for the rights of others, anger is a positive force. These people and organizations changed the world with their anger:

- Dr. Martin Luther King's leadership in the civil rights movement

  Susan B. Anthony's fight for women's right to vote

- Nelson Mandela's fight against apartheid MADD (Mothers

  Against Drunk Driving) SAVE (Students Against Violence

  Everywhere)

Choose one to read about, and tell how anger was channeled into somethingpositive.

_____

_____

_____

_____

_____

_____

_____

_____

_____

_____

Exercise 13 chilling out

---

for you to know

When you are angry, choosing an Exercise that helps you calm down will keep your anger from getting the best of you.

Ethan's younger brother Ryan was a pain in the neck. Whenever Ethan was watching television, Ryan wanted to change the channel. If Ethan was talking on the phone, Ryan would interrupt. He would borrow Ethan's CDs without askingand then forget where he had put them.

One evening at dinner, Ethan was just about to take a slice of watermelon for dessert when Ryan reached across and grabbed the last piece. That was it! Ethan shoved his brother, who started to cry. Their mom sent both boys away from the table.

Later that evening, she knocked on Ethan's door and asked if they could talk. She said, "Ethan, I know that Ryan often bugs you, but shoving him is not acceptable. Let's talk about what you can do to chill out when you feel angry with him." Together, Ethan and his mom came up with this list:

- *Talk to someone.Take a time-out. Text a friend.*

- *Pound on a pillow.Play an instrument.*

- *Listen to relaxing music.Go for a bike ride.*

- *Play basketball.Read a book.*

- *Draw.*

- *Write in a journal.*

The next time Ethan found himself getting angry with Ryan, he simply stretchedout on the sofa with his iPod. Pretty soon, he could hardly remember what had made him so angry!

for you to do

Think about situations that often make you angry. When these situations arise, tell how you can chill out instead of exploding.

I get angry when _____

_____

I can chill out by _____

_____

I get angry when _____

_____

I can chill out by _____

_____

I get angry when _____

_____

I can chill out by _____

_____

... and more to do!

Using old magazines and newspapers, cut out pictures that remind you of your favorite ways to chill out. For example, if swimming helps you chill out, you might add a picture of a swimmer or a lake. Paste the pictures on a blank piece of paper or cardboard. Put your chill-out poster where you are most likely to find it helpful — perhaps in a notebook, on your desk, or in your locker.

Exercise 14writing

---

for you to know

When you hold in your anger, it is likely to build. Expressing your feelings is an important first step toward coping with them, and writing is a great way to do that. How well you write or whether you follow grammar rules is not important in this type of writing. What is important is getting your feelings out.

Exploring your emotions is like dumping out a puzzle and sorting through the pieces. At first, the task may seem overwhelming. But once you begin to match up some pieces, the rest begin to fall into place. Think of writing as a way to help you sort through the puzzle pieces of life.

If you've never expressed your feelings this way before, a great way to start is by writing a letter to yourself. You can pretend that you're writing to a close friend whom you trust with your life. Silly as it may sound, writing a letter to yourself lets you explore your thoughts and feelings. You have no one to impress, so you can be honest about what you want to change about your behavior.

for you to do

Write a letter to yourself. Include things that you are unhappy about, disappointed with, or want to change. Talk about why angerhas been a problem for you and why you want to handle it differently.

When you have finished your letter, photocopy it and place the copy in an envelope. Put it somewhere safe and plan to open it in six months. You may besurprised at the changes that you've made!

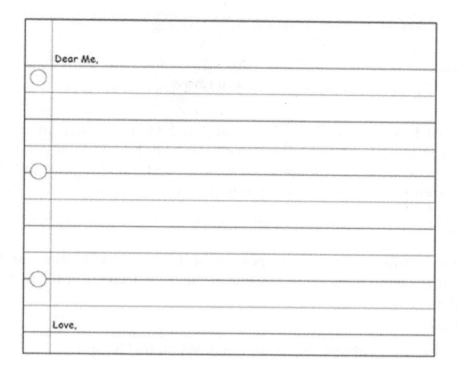

Dear Me,

Love,

... and more to do!

Journaling is a great way to help you cope with your anger. You can make a habit of writing down your thoughts and feelings rather than bottling them up, especially when something is bothering you. Expressing yourself in writing can help you examine whatever is bugging you. Then you can develop a plan to handle the situation rather than reacting impulsively, which often leads to negative consequences.

Exercise 15 laughing at anger

for you to know

Humor is a great way to defuse anger. Not only can it improve a tense situation, but it's also good for your health! A good laugh reduces your level of stress hormones and boosts your level of endorphins, which are hormones that give you a sense of well-being.

Anger and humor are polar opposites, so it's hard to be angry and laugh at the same time. Look at some of the ways that laughter and anger can affect you.

Laughter:

makes you forget about your anger makes you feel happy

gives you a great stomach workout makes others want to be with you decreases tension

Anger:

makes you focus on what you're mad about makes you unhappy

causes your heart to beat faster hurts your relationships with others makes you tense

A situation that makes you angry is likely to have a different outcome depending on whether you allow your anger to escalate or your sense of humor to take over. Many episodes of anger are actually funny, if you can step away from what has happened long enough to notice. So next time you get angry, stop and ask yourself, "What's funny about this situation?" Chances are you'll find some humor if you just look for it.

for you to do *Jake's dad had reminded him twice to take out the garbage. Jake knew he had to do it, but he was in the middle of a video game and didn't want to be interrupted. At his dad's third reminder, Jake stormed into the kitchen and grabbed the lid off the trash can. He jerked* *the garbage bag out with so much force that it burst open and trash flew across the kitchen floor. To make things even worse, Jake slipped on the remains ofthat evening's dinner! When his father came into the kitchen to see what all the commotion was about, he found Jake lying on the floor surrounded by trash.*

Write an ending that shows what might have happened if Jake continued to allowhis anger to take over.

_____

_____

_____

_____

Next, write an ending that shows Jake finding some humor in what happened.

_____

_____

_____

_____

... and more to do!

Think of a time when you reacted to a situation with anger.Describe the situation and what you did.

_____

_____

_____

_____

_____

_____

_____

Imagine you had been able to find humor in this situation, and rewrite yourexperience showing how the outcome would have been different.

_____

_____

_____

_____

_____

_____

_____

Exercise 16
taking a mental vacation

for you to know

Having a special place where you feel comfortable and relaxed can help when you're upset. Even if you can't actually visit it, just going there in your imagination can help you clear your head and calm yourself.

Kayla was having a terrible day. All of her friends had turned against her at school because of a rumor that wasn't even true. She thought, "Whoever started that rumor is going to regret ever mentioning my name!" She couldn't wait untilshe got home. She just wanted to go to her room and close out the world.

TJ's girlfriend had just broken up with him over the weekend, and she was already going out with another guy. He was furious with her and upset that everyone would realize she had dumped him. If he could only disappear for a while … maybe go to the beach where his problems would seem so small compared to the ocean. He had a lot of good memories of times at the beach and always felt relaxed when he was there.

Have you ever felt like Kayla or TJ? Do you have a place you like to escape to when things aren't going well? You may not always be able to go to that special place right away. That's okay; you can still take a mental vacation and just imagine being there.

for you to do

Imagine you're a travel agent setting up a website that offers "Emotional Getaway" vacation packages. Write the description of your favorite spot for calming down. Include how you feel when youare there.

_____

_____

_____

_____

... and more to do!

In the space below, draw yourself in your mental vacation spot. The next time you feel overwhelmed by a situation that makes you angry, imagine yourself being there.

Exercise 17 releasing anger symbolically

> **for you to know**
>
> Holding anger inside is harmful for you but you can find ways to release your feelings symbolically.

Imagery and symbolism can help people cope with things that bother them in life. For example, parents in the Ojibwa Nation would hang dream catchers above their children's beds. The dream catcher was thought to trap bad dreams in the web that formed its center; good dreams would be allowed to flow down itsfeathers to the sleeping child. Then, in the morning, the sunlight would destroy the bad dreams that were caught in the web.

Another example of symbolic imagery is the "Wish-Giving Tree" in Shenzhen,China. Legend has it that in 1410, Tianhou, goddess of the sea, miraculously rescued the explorer Admiral Zheng. Tianhou later appeared to Zheng in a dreamand instructed him to build a temple in her honor. A tree that was planted in the temple's courtyard still stands today, and people write down their problems on red slips of paper, which they attach to the tree.

This tree or a dream catcher don't literally take away problems, but they do release them symbolically, which is a wonderful way to cope.

Here are other symbolic ways to help you manage your anger:

- Write a letter to someone you are angry at. Tell that person what youreally think and then tear up the letter.

- Imagine that a pillow is a person you are mad at and hit the

  pillow. Skip pebbles across a pond, letting an angry thought go

  with each one.

- Shoot baskets or kick a soccer ball toward a goal, imagining an angry
- situation with each shot.

- Write down your angry thoughts on a sheet of paper and then paint overthem.

for you to do

This Exercise will help you symbolically release angry feelings you have been holding in. You'll need a balloon, small strips of paper, and something to write with.

On each strip of paper, write down something that made you really angry and that you haven't let go of. Next, roll each strip tightly and place it inside the balloon. Then blow air into the balloon, and as you do, focus on all the things you wrote down. After you have blown the balloon full of anger, hold the top of it closed. Take some deep breaths, say good-bye to everything the balloon is holding inside, and let it go. Watch as your worries sail across the room and areforever released.

... and more to do!

How did you feel physically after releasing your anger?

_____

_____

How did you feel emotionally?

_____

_____

Are there other feelings that you'd like to release (for example, sadness over a breakup with a girlfriend or boyfriend, stress over a family problem, or fear of failure in school)? Write them here.

_____

_____

Have you ever tried any of the symbolic releases mentioned earlier in thisExercise? If so, what did you do, and how did you feel after doing it?

Exercise 18 relaxation techniques

---

for you to know

When you get angry, your body reacts. Your heart may race; your breathing may speed up; your muscles may tense.

These reactions make it hard for you to think clearly and get control of your anger, so knowing how to relax is important.

Managing anger becomes easier when you are relaxed. You can use these helpfultechniques when you want to calm yourself.

- Find a quiet location and get into a comfortable position. Starting at yourtoes and working all the way up to your head, tense your entire body, including your arms and hands. Hold that tension for a minute. Take a deep breath and let it out as you slowly release the tension from your head all the way to your toes so that you end up feeling like a rag doll. Repeat two or three times.

- Go to a spot where you won't be distracted or interrupted. Close your eyes and start to take slow, deep breaths, filling your lungs completely full of air and releasing it. Repeat several times until you feel yourself beginning to relax. Deep breathing increases the flow of oxygen to yourbrain, which helps you focus.

- Take a warm bath or shower and imagine washing away all of your anger. The water will help to relax your muscles.

- Read a book. Reading is a wonderful way to escape the world for a while. When you come back to reality, you'll be able to think more clearly.

- Take a nap. When you sleep, your body totally relaxes and goes into a meditative state. You'll wake up feeling more refreshed and ready to handle whatever is troubling you.

for you to do

We all have different ideas about what is relaxing. One person might think of a beach, a park, a cell phone, and an ice skating rink; another might picture a fishing rod, a book, a pair of running shoes, and an iPod. Using old magazines or newspapers, find images that represent your idea of relaxation. On a separate piece of paper, make a collage of these images. Put your collage in your room as a reminder of ways to relax when you're angry.

... and more to do!

Write down three activities that are your favorite ways to relax.

1. _____

2. _____

3. _____

Write down three new relaxation activities you would like to try.

1. _____

2. _____

3. _____

Which Exercise do you think will be most effective in helping you calm down?

_____

After you have tried one or more of your relaxation activities a few times, tell how they worked.

_____

_____

_____

Exercise 19

handling anger constructively

---

for you to know

Most of us can remember times when we regretted how we handled situations that made us angry. Instead of finding yourself in that position over and over, you can prepare yourself by thinking in advance about how you might react.

John had really done it this time. He was engrossed in his video game and had almost made it to a level he'd never reached before. Suddenly Cody, his five-year-old brother, charged into the room, flying his toy Stealth Bomber, and tripped, pulling the power cable from the wall. That did it! John picked up his video remote and hurled it at Cody, breaking a vase in the process. Cody started to cry. As John heard his mother coming toward them, he thought, "It was all Cody's fault, that little brat. Now I'm really in for it."

His mom came in and checked that Cody was okay. Then she looked around and noticed the vase. She asked John what had happened. When he explained, she said "John, no more video games today, and you'll have to clean up this mess. I know you were angry that Cody ruined your game. But you might have hurt your brother, and you broke my favorite vase. What else could you have done instead of throwing the remote at Cody?"

John thought about it for a while. Then he said, "I guess I could have closed my door. Or I could have told Cody how angry I was instead of throwing something at him."

for you to do

Read each scenario and respond to the questions.

Janet really needed to pull up her biology grade. As she was taking notes in biology class, Kyle kept throwing little pieces of paper at her. "What a pain," she thought. "If he does it once more, that's it!" As their teacher went on to describe the process of photosynthesis, Kyle pelted Janet with another piece of paper. Janet turned around in her chair, got in Kyle's face, and started to yell. She was escorted from class to the principal's office.

What are some of the consequences that Janet may face?_____

_____

_____

_____

What are some of the dangers in Janet's actions?_____

_____

_____

_____

How could Janet have handled the situation more appropriately? _____

_____

_____

_____

Tim had gotten his license six months earlier and he already had two traffic violations. As he started to change lanes, another driver pulled right in front of him and Tim almost rear-ended the car. "I've got to get by this dude!" he thought. He hit the accelerator, pulled around, and built up to 60 mph — in a 45 mph zone! Before Tim could slow down, police lights were flashing behind him.

What are some of the consequences that Tim may face?

_____

_____

_____

What are some of the dangers in Tim's actions?

_____

_____

_____

How could Tim have handled the situation more appropriately?

_____

_____

_____

… and more to do!

Tell about a time when you were angry and reacted poorly.

_____

_____

_____

What were some of the consequences you faced?

_____

_____

_____

What were some of the dangers of your actions?

_____

_____

_____

What did you learn from this situation?

_____

_____

_____

Knowing what you know now, how could you have handled the situationdifferently?

_____

_____

_____

Exercise 20 anger contract

---

for you to know

When you're caught up in anger, it's hard to tell people howto help you, so it's a good idea to have a plan to put in place before it happens. Letting others know that you are working on your anger and what they can do to help is a big step toward change.

Signing a contract is a way of making a commitment. It is like promising yourself that you will work hard to change your behavior. Sharing this commitment with other people — friends, family members, teachers, or other important adults — will help you honor it.

The first step is to decide what cues you will use to let these people know when you are getting angry. Your contract will also identify places where you can go to cool down and let others know what to do — and what not to do — when you get angry.

for you to do

Anger Contract

I am working on controlling my anger. As part of this change, I am making a commitment that you can help mewith.

When I feel myself getting angry, I will give you one of these cues: 1._____ 2._____ 3._____

If you notice that I am getting ready to lose my temper, please let me know by using one of these signals: 1._____ 2._____ 3._____

I will then go to one of these places to cool down. 1._2.

_____ 3._____

Please do not do the following things. They only frustrate me more.

When I have had a chance to cool down, I will return in a calmer frame of mind.

Signed by_____ Date _____

---

1. _____
2. _____
3. _____

... and more to do!

Once you have drawn up your contract, think about whom you will ask to help you. Some possibilities include your parents, teachers, counselor, coach, siblings, and close friends. Write their names here.

_____

_____

_____

Make several copies of your contract. Keep one for yourself and give the others to those you have chosen. Check off each name when you give that person a copy of your contract.

Exercise 21
taking responsibility for your own actions

---

for you to know

When something goes wrong, it's much easier to blame others than to admit that we played a role in causing the problem. But blaming others doesn't resolve conflict; it just makes it worse. Before laying the blame on others, ask yourself, "What role do I have in this?" Once you learn to take responsibility for your own actions, you'll be less likely to push your anger onto someone else.

Tavaris knew that it was against the rules to have his cell phone at school, but he just couldn't resist sporting his new high-tech phone. He was sitting in Social Studies class when Joe asked to see his phone. Tavaris reached into his pocket and passed it back. As Joe was playing around with the phone, their teacher walked up. He took the phone and told Tavaris that his parents would have to come to school to pick it up. He also gave Tavaris detention for having a cell phone in class. Tavaris was ticked at Joe. It was all Joe's fault!

Ever been in a situation similar to this? It's clear that it wasn't all Joe's fault that Tavaris lost his phone or had to stay after school, but when you're angry it's easy to blame someone else for what happened. Tavaris needs to step back and look at the big picture. He can begin by asking: "How did I get myself into this?"

Nicole hated babysitting her little sister, Katie. Katie was constantly getting into everything. Nicole never could get anything done with her around. On this particular day, Nicole was supposed to be watching Katie while their parents were out. While Nicole was on the phone with her boyfriend, Katie got hold of their mother's red lipstick and played Picasso all over the living-room walls. When their parents got home, they were very angry with Nicole. She was placed on restriction for a month. Nicole thought, "This isn't fair! It isn't right that I'm the one getting in trouble. I didn't do it!"

Life ever treated you unfairly? In Nicole's case, rather than blaming someoneelse for the problem, she feels as though she's the one being blamed.

for you to do

Help Tavaris and Nicole step back and look at their contributions tothe situations.

What role did Tavaris play in causing the problem?

_____

_____

_____

How could he have taken responsibility for his own actions?

_____

_____

_____

What role did Nicole play in causing the problem?

_____

_____

How could she have taken responsibility for her own actions?

_____

_____

_____

... and more to do!

Briefly describe a time when you blamed another person forsomething you did.

_____

_____

_____

Have you ever been accused of something that you didn't do? What happened?

_____

_____

_____

Why do you think it's easier to blame others for your problems than to acceptresponsibility?

_____

_____

_____

The next time you find yourself either blaming or being blamed, what can youdo to keep from getting angry?

_____

_____

_____

Exercise 22 keeping perspective

---

for you to know

We all overreact to situations at times, but when it happens frequently it can lead to big problems. Keeping perspective means recognizing when you're blowing things out of proportion. You can then change your response so that the situation doesn't get out of control.

Katherine was having one of the worst days of her life. She had totally forgotten that her term paper was due, not to mention that she had overslept and was late to school. "Is this day ever going to end?" she thought. On her way to her next class, she noticed her friends Leslie and Jasmine standing next to her locker, looking mischievous. "What's up, guys?" she asked. "Nothing," they responded innocently and smiled at each other.

When Katherine opened her locker, her books were missing. "I am so not in the mood for this!" she said. She hit the locker, threw her backpack across the hall, and slammed her locker shut. She made such a commotion that everyone was staring and teachers ran into the hallway to see what was going on.

Leslie looked at Katherine. "What's your deal? Here are your books. We were just playing with you." Both Leslie and Jasmine walked off, leaving Katherine humiliated as everyone watched.

Ever had a Katherine moment? Odds are you have. It usually happens when you're having a bad day and any little thing can push you over the edge. Here's the good news: you can keep situations in perspective and stop yourself from overreacting.

To avoid blowing things out of proportion, Katherine could have tried the following:

- **Known her feelings:** Katherine knew she was in a bad mood. She could either have avoided her mischievous friends and gone to her locker later or just walked away when she opened the empty locker.

- **Spoken her feelings:** Rather than making a spectacle of herself, Katherine could have simply told her friends, "Look, I'm having a reallybad day, and I am so not in the mood for this. Can you just give me backmy books?"

- **Joked it off:** Since her friends were playing around, Katherine could have played back by saying something like, "Okay, that's funny, and you got me. Now I really need my books, so I'm not late for another class." This approach might have resulted in getting her books back quicker without an audience watching.

for you to do

Briefly describe a time when you blew a situation out of proportion.

_____

_____

_____

What were you thinking?

_____

_____

_____

What was the outcome of the situation?

_____

_____

_____

What could you do differently the next time you're faced with a similar situation?

_____

_____

_____

… and more to do!

How can being aware of your thoughts and feelings keep you from overreacting?

_____

_____

_____

If you repeatedly overreact to situations, how do you think it will affect yourrelationships with others?

_____

_____

_____

What are some consequences you have faced because of overreacting? (Forexample,   have you lost   friends   or

_____

_____

_____

Exercise 23 getting the facts

---

for you to know

Assuming that you know what others are thinking and feeling is a slippery slope that can get you into deep trouble. Rather than responding to situations with anger, it is important to be sure you have the facts straight.

Kristen had a really bad crush on Cole, a new kid at school. When she told her friend Lisa how much she liked Cole, Lisa asked, "Do you want me to do a little matchmaking?" "No! Don't say a word!" Kristen said. Lisa agreed that she wouldn't.

Finally it was time for lunch, and Kristen was looking forward to seeing Cole. When she walked into the cafeteria, she saw Lisa talking to Cole. When Lisa and Cole spotted Kristen from across the cafeteria, they smiled and waved. Kristin shot Lisa a dirty look. "What?" Lisa mouthed. "You know what!" Kristen mouthed back. She stomped across the cafeteria and in front of everyone gave Lisa a piece of her mind.

In this example, Kristen reacted based on her belief that Lisa had told Cole her feelings, but she didn't actually have all the information. Have you ever assumed you knew what was going on in a situation when in reality you didn't have a clue?

When you catch yourself making assumptions, do this:

- Say, "Stop it!" Every time you catch yourself thinking you know whatsomeone else is thinking, tell yourself to stop.

- Think positively. Think of how you may be misreading the situation. Tryto see other sides of the story rather than focusing on what you "think"

- you know.

- Realize that not everyone thinks as you do. What you think may be quitedifferent from reality. Seek out the facts before you react.

- Ask yourself, "Am I jumping to conclusions?" You may not have all the information you need to make a decision. Do you react to information you've received from others rather than the person you're in conflict with?

- Ask for the truth. Go directly to the person and ask what's going on. What's the worst thing that will happen?

for you to do

Rewrite Kristen's story using the suggestions given earlier.

_____

_____

_____

_____

… and more to do!

Have you ever made wrong assumptions about a situation? Tell what happened.

_____

What happened when you found out that you were wrong?

_____

_____

_____

_____

_____

What might have happened if you had gotten all the facts?

Exercise 24 stages of anger

---

for you to know

Anger builds in stages. By understanding the progression of your anger, you can learn to quickly identify when you are becoming agitated and head it off before it gets out of control.

Alex's story can show you how anger progresses.

1. Your anger button gets pushed.

   Alex was getting ready for his big soccer game. He looked at the clock; it was 5:15. He was supposed to be at the field in fifteen minutes, and no one was home to drive him. "Where are my parents?" he thought. He tried calling, but no one answered. Every minute, Alex became more agitated.

Can you guess what Alex's button pusher is? If you guessed "being late," you're right!

2. Your thinking gets distorted.

   While Alex was anxiously waiting for his parents to arrive, he kept thinking, "By the time I get there, the game's going to be half over and all the guys will be ticked at me! I'll probably be kicked off the team."

Anger tends to distort how people think about situations. Notice how Alex assumed the worst-case scenario and blew things out of proportion. Other common distortions include blaming others and misinterpreting events.

3. Your feelings take over and you react.

   When his dad pulled into the driveway and honked for Alex at 5:40, Alex rushed out of the house. His face was red, and he slammed his hand against the car. He glared at his father and shouted, "I can't believe you did this! The coach is going to get on me, and it's all your fault!"

Notice how Alex's feelings have taken control of his behavior. He was worried that he might be kicked off the team; he was embarrassed about facing the team and coach; he was hurt that his parents hadn't even thought to call him. Most of all, he was angry that he was going to be late.

for you to do

Once Alex's button was pushed, his anger quickly progressed. In the space below, write a new ending for his story. How could he have thought differently? How else could he have reacted?

_____

_____

_____

… and more to do!

Think of a time when you were angry. Describe each stage of your anger. Then go back and circle the key words that indicate you were in that stage.

Stage 1. Your anger button gets pushed. (What really set you

_____

_____

_____

Stage 2. Your thinking gets distorted. (How might you have misinterpreted the situation, blamed others, or blown things out of proportion?)

_____

_____

_____

Stage 3. Your feelings take over and you react. (What other feeling went along with your anger?) _____

_____

_____

What do you think would be the best outcome of learning to change yourreaction to anger?

_____

_____

_____

Exercise 25perception

Mallory and Casey were at the movies. Mallory saw their friend Sarah sitting nearby with Noah, the boy Casey really liked. The two were whispering, their heads close together. Mallory couldn't believe what she was seeing. Were Sarah and Noah an item? How could Sarah? Casey's birthday was just around the corner. What a birthday present this was going to be!

Casey also noticed Sarah and Noah whispering together. "What are those two up to?" she thought. "They seem to be planning something. I wonder if it has to do with my birthday."

Mallory and Casey both saw the same thing but came up with different conclusions. Has that ever happened to you?

for you to do

Do you see this glass as half-full or half-empty? Changing the way you look at a situation can change the way you react. On the left, write down negative thoughts you have had about situations. On the right, reframe your thoughts so that they are positive.

Negative Thoughts

My friend didn't call me.
She must be mad.

_____
_____
_____
_____
_____

Positive Thoughts

She's probably been busy.
I'll call her.

_____
_____
_____
_____
_____

... and more to do!

Look at the pictures below. See if you can find a friend to do these activities with you.

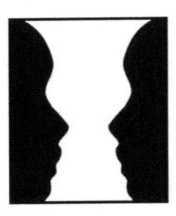 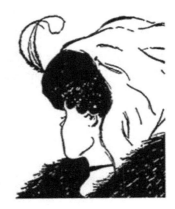

In the picture on the left, do you see a vase or the profiles of two people? On the right, do you see a young woman or an old woman? If you can you see both, notice which one you see first. Show these pictures to a friend. Do you both see them the same way? If not, does that make one of you wrong?

Just as with these images, in life there are two or more sides to every story. Frequently we accuse others of being wrong simply because they don't see things the way we do. Wouldn't it be great if we could see all sides before we react?

Exercise 26 weighing the options

For you to know

Some decisions are easier than others. Some don't require much thought at all, while others cause a lot of stress. One thing is certain: Decisions made in anger are likely to be impulsive and usually don't have good outcomes.

That's why it's important to weigh your options before you react.

You will make many decisions in life. Some will be small, such as what to wear for the dance or which movie to see. Some will be big: Do you get into the car with your best friend even though he's been drinking? Do you go out with that cute guy even though he's got a bad reputation?

When you are angry, it is much harder to exercise good judgment when you have a choice to make. By making it a habit to think before you act, you can learn to react thoughtfully rather than giving in to anger.

for you to do

Several of Jeremiah's friends told him that a kid named Cody wanted to fight him after school. Cody had been running his mouth about Jeremiah since day one, and Jeremiah was sick of it. He wanted to finish this once and for all but wasn't sure he wanted to fight. So before he made a choice, he listed the costs and benefits involved. His list included these things:

- I might be expelled from school. I may have to go to court.

- I could hurt Cody badly.
- My parents will ground me for life. Cody could hurt me.

- I could get charged with assault.

- It will feel good to shut Cody up once and for all.Cody will learn

  not to mess with me.

- Others will leave me alone.

Help Jeremiah weigh his options—to fight or not—by deciding whether eachitem above is a cost or a benefit. Then write them in the correct column.

Costs of Fighting	Benefits of Fighting

Tell what decision you think Jeremiah made, and why.

_____

_____

... and more to do!

Think of a decision you have to make. Record what the decision isand weigh the costs and the benefits.

Decision to Be Made	
Decision:	
Costs	Benefits

Each time you have a decision to make, weigh your options by listing the costs and benefits. Looking at a decision that way often helps the answer become clear.

Excercise 27
the abc model of anger

for you to know

Learning to change your thoughts about frustrating situations will help you control your anger. Some counselors use a simple approach called the ABC model to teach people how to change their thoughts about a situation.

Here's how the ABC model works: A = Activating event (the situation that makes you angry) You were working on your term paper and took a brief break. While you were away from the computer, your brother went to check his MySpace page. The lights flickered, and when you got back to your computer, your last hour of work was gone.

B = Beliefs about the event

> Beliefs can be rational and irrational. Rational beliefs are accurate interpretations of the event; for example, "I lost my work because of a power dip." Irrational beliefs involve distorted thoughts, which were explored in earlier activities. For example:

- *It was all his fault!* (blaming others rather than taking responsibility; seeExercise 21.)

- *I'll probably fail – if I ever get to finish!* (blowing things out of proportion rather than keeping perspective; see Exercise 22.)

- *He always messes around with my things.* (making assumptions ratherthan getting the facts; see Exercise 23.)

C = Consequences

> You throw a book at your brother. You yell at him, telling him that youhate him and wish he had never been born!

The next step is to look at your beliefs and decide whether they are rational ornot. If they are not, you follow these three steps:

4. Dispute your beliefs. Think: *"Maybe it was an accident. It's not like*

he

5. *has any control over the power. I should have saved my work. Maybe he didn't know I was using the computer."*

6. Set goals to avoid similar situations in the future. Decide: *"I want to protect my work as best as I can. I want to be on good terms with my brother."*

7. Create a plan to support your goals. Plan: *"I'll set the computer up for automatic save. I'll tell others when I'm working on something important. I'll apologize for the way I reacted and try not to automatically blame my brother."*

for you to do

Now it's your turn to put the ABC model to work. Think of a recent situation that made you angry. Use the model to help you work through your thoughts and actions.

What was the activating event (the situation that made you angry)?

_____

_____

What were your irrational beliefs about the event?

_____

_____

What were the consequences of those beliefs?

_____

_____

How can you dispute your beliefs?

_____

_____

What goals can you set to avoid similar situations in the future?

_____

_____

Create a plan to support your goals.

_____

_____

... and more to do!

The next time you catch yourself getting angry about something, use the ABC model to help you work through the situation. The model will help you to look at things from another perspective and change your irrational beliefs. You can create a visual reminder to use this model by making an index card with the steps on it. Keep this card in a place that is easily accessible so you can get to it quickly. Soon you'll be able to put the steps in place without even needing to refer to the card.

Exercise 28 coping with conflict

for you to know

Some reactions make it easier to resolve a conflict, while others make it harder. Being aware of your own style can help you learn to respond in a positive way. And since people react to conflict in different ways, it is also helpful if you can recognize others' styles.

Here are some common ways people react to conflict.

The Competitor: It's your way or the highway. You're bound and determined to win, no matter the cost. You blame and accuse others of being wrong. You're always right. You're going to get the final word in, if it's the last thing you do!

The Doormat: You let others take advantage of you. Saying no has never been easy for you, so you become a doormat for others to walk on, which makes you angry. But you won't say or do anything because you don't want to make anyone mad at you.

The Bolter: In difficult situations, you bolt! You avoid conflict at all costs, no matter how angry a situation has made you. You tell yourself that there's nothing you can do about it. You rarely find a solution for your problems. You just bottle them up. Needless to say, you have a lot of unfinished business.

The Team Builder: When you have a conflict with someone, you stay focused on what happened rather than launching an attack on the other person. You try to resolve the conflict by meeting in the middle, or compromising. If you can't compromise, you agree to disagree and move on.

Can you guess which approach is the most effective? If you guessed the Team Builder, you're right! Team builders try to understand a situation before reacting. By using good listening and communication skills, they are more likely to get others to listen to how they feel, making it easier to resolve a conflict.

for you to do

Read these examples, and decide which approach to conflict is being used. Write your answer in the space provided. Answers are listed at the bottom of the page.

1. Math had always been Jan's hardest subject. She constantly struggled in class and didn't understand her homework. Now her dad was on her case again about her math grades. "There is no excuse for your doing so poorly, Jan. I am sick and tired of getting calls from your math teacher. What do you have to say for yourself?" he yelled. She wanted to tell him how much trouble math was for her, but she was afraid that he would just get angrier! "Nothing, Dad. I'll try harder. May I be excused? I have some homework that I need to do," she replied. With that, Jan made a quick dash for her room. As soon as she was inside, she shut the door and leaned against it. "Oh, he makes me so angry!" she thought.

    _____

2. Matt's best friend, Jacob, really hurt him this time. Matt had told Jacob for months how he really liked Emily. How could Jacob have asked her out on a date? Matt felt angry but he was worried that if he said something to Jacob, he might lose his best friend. Maybe it wasn't worth saying anything. Emily and Jacob would probably make a better couple anyway. _____

3. Carrie caught her mom reading her diary. How could she? Carrie took a deep breath and said, "Mom, why are you reading my diary? I feel like you don't trust me, and that hurts my feelings." Together, Carrie and her mom talked about privacy and trust. By the end of the conversation, Carrie's mom agreed to respect her space. In return, Carrie agreed to share more about what was going on in her life with her mom.

    _____

4. Tara and Jamie were in a heated argument over their plans to go shopping. Jamie wanted to ask the new girl at school to join them, but Tara wanted to keep it to just the two of them. The bell rang to

signal thatlunch period was over, and as Tara got up to leave, she turned back to Jamie and said, "You're such a do-gooder!" That did it for Jamie. She gotin Tara's face and screamed, "Maybe so, but you're a snob—a super snob!" Then she stormed off before Tara could say another word.

_____

1. Bolter; 2. Doormat; 3. Team Builder; 4. Competitor Next, choose the Bolter,the Competitor, or the Doormat example and rewrite it using the Team Builder style.

_____

_____

_____

_____

_____ ... and more to do!

_____

_____

_____

_____

_____

_____

_____

_____

_____

Think about how you usually react to conflict. Put a 1 next to the style you are most likely to use and continuing ranking the other styles from 2 to 4.

_____The Competitor

_____The Doormat

_____The Bolter

_____ The Team Builder If you use a different approach to conflict, describe it here.

_____

_____

_____

Ask several people who know you well how they think you most often react to conflict. Write down their responses here. Do most agree with the style you ranked first?

_____

_____

_____

Tell about a conflict you recently had. How could you have resolved it using the Team Builder style?

_____

_____

_____

_____

Exercise 29 using I-messages

for you to know

I-messages express how you feel without making others feel that they are to blame. Learning to use I-messages instead of you-messages is a simple but important way to improve your communication skills.

You-messages focus on what other people have done in a way that makes them feel as though they are being attacked. These messages often include words that put people on the defensive, like "should," "always," "must," "ought to," and "never." When you start finger pointing and making accusations, people are likely to stop listening to you. Instead, they focus on what they are going to say in response to your attack.

An I-message tells what you feel, what the person has done to make you feel that way, and why you feel the way you do. By using I-messages instead of you- messages, you can decrease tension in a conflict. The other person is less apt to feel defensive, and it will be easier for the two of you to work out a solution to whatever situation has caused the anger.

Here are two examples:

1. You are angry with a friend who usually eats lunch with you but has been sitting at a different table all week.
2. You-message: You always ignore me!
3. I-message: I feel hurt when you don't sit with me at lunch because it makes me think that you don't want to be my friend.

4. You have been trying to tell your friend about a problem at home, but she keeps responding to each new text message she gets.
5. You-message: You never listen to me!
6. I-message: I feel angry when you keep texting while I'm trying to talk to you because it makes me think that you don't care about what I am saying.

Which message would you be more willing to listen to?

for you to do

Now it's your turn to try these messages. For each situation, write down how you would respond using a you-message. Next, change that response to a more helpful I-message.

The boy sitting behind you in class is using his pencil as a drumstick.

You-message: You_____.

I-message: I feel_____when you
_____because_____.

Your friend totally humiliates you in front of the class by telling everyone whoyou have a crush on.

You-message: You_____.

I-message: I feel_____when you
_____because_____.

Your group is supposed to present their project in class today. You find out thatyou are the only one who did any of the work.

You-message: You_____.

I-message: I feel_____when you
_____because_____.

Your mother comes home from work. You've been cleaning the house buthaven't gotten to your room yet. She accuses you of not doing anything.

You-message: You_____.

I-message: I feel_____when you
_____because_____.

Another kid trips you as you are walking down the hall.

You-message: You_____.

I-message: I feel_____when you
_____because_____.

... and more to do!

For one week, keep a tally of all of the times that you use you- messages. Notice whether they include the words "should," "always," "must," "ought to," or "never." On the table below, make a check mark for each time that you use a you-message that day. Next, in columns 3 through 7, place a check mark for each defensive word that you use in your you-message.

	You-Messages	Should	Always	Must	Ought To	Never
Monday						
Tuesday						
Wednesday						
Thursday						
Friday						
Saturday						
Sunday						
Total						

Add up the accusatory messages. Which of the statements did you use mostfrequently?

_____

Now that you are aware of using this language, how do you plan to change it?

_____

_____

_____

Exercise 30 good listening

for you to know

By using I-messages to express your own feelings and building good listening skills that help you understand how others are feeling, you can defuse anger-provoking situations.

Communication is an important part of working through anger, and being a good listener is an important part of communication. Listening well helps you connect to the person you are upset with so that you can understand each other better.

Good listeners share these characteristics:

They pay attention to the person who is speaking. They keep eye contact.

They show interest by nodding or by smiling at appropriate times.

They make sure that they understand what has been said by repeating it in their own words. For example, a good listener might say, "Do you mean that ...?"

They let the other person finish his or her thoughts without

interrupting. They ask questions if anything is not clear when the speaker

has finished.

for you to do

Think of a time when you were a good listener.

What was the other person talking about?

_____

What did you do to show that person you were listening?

How did that person react?

Now think of a time when someone listened well to you. What were you talking about?

How could you tell that the other person was listening carefully?

How did being listened to make you feel?

How can listening help defuse anger?

… and more to do!

How often do you really listen to others? One great place to practice your listening skills is with a close friend. The next time you're with a friend, ask him or her a question. Then sit back and just listen.

Did you listen well?_____Yes_____No If yes, which of the suggestions listedearlier did you follow?

If no, what did you do that showed you were not listening well?

What will you do differently in the future?

Exercise 31 complimenting others

for you to know

Being complimented makes most people feel good on the inside. On the other hand, being torn down is likely to make someone feel horrible and often leads to angry feelings.

Amanda was in a very playful mood in gym class. She started to sing. Jenna, who was having a really bad day, quickly had enough of Amanda's singing and called out, "Girl, you can't sing! Have you ever heard yourself? Whoever said you could was deaf! Just shut up!"

How do you think Amanda felt after that verbal assault? She was probably embarrassed, hurt, and maybe a little angry. It's easy to use words to tear peopledown. But have you ever tried using words to build them up? You'll get a completely different reaction. Don't you feel good when someone pays you a compliment, like, "You look nice today" or "Hey, those are cool shoes"? You can do the same for others!

for you to do

Put a check next to each sentence you can use to compliment someone. Put an X next to those sentences that would tear someone down.

- Your help was really important.I am very proud of you.

- That's stupid.

- You never do anything right.You did a great job!

- You aced the test.

- You screw up all the time.You are really nice.

- I couldn't have done this without you.You're so lazy.

- I can't stand listening to you. You're hopeless.

- You're a great friend. You always listen.

- What a whiner you are! I can't tell you anything. You're so trustworthy.

- You're a nerd.

... and more to do!

Think of positive things people have told you that made you feel good. Write their statements in the speech balloons below.

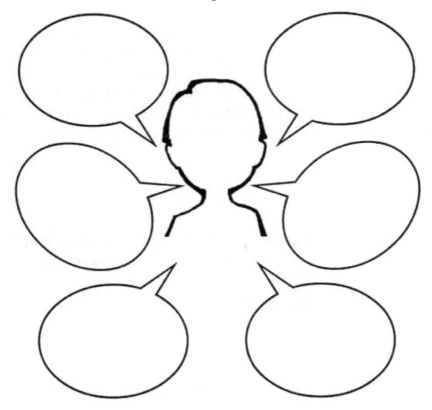

Exercise 32 body language

The idea that you can communicate without speaking might seem strange, but it's true. Most communication between people takes place without words; it is based on body language. Your body language, also called nonverbal communication, is made up of your gestures, facial expressions, posture, and even your tone of voice. This language lets others know what you are feeling.

Look at some of the ways people use body language to express their negative feelings:

- rolling their eyes plugging their earscrossing their armsglaring

- sighing

- clenching their fistsbiting their lips gritting their teeth

- tapping their feet impatientlypointing a finger at someone

- Not all body language communicates negative feelings. Here are some examplesof positive messages:

- waving hello smiling hugging blowing a kiss

- patting someone on the backclapping

- giving someone a thumbs-upnodding in agreement

for you to do

For an entire day, notice how people communicate without words. Write down the body language you observe, the situation it occurs in, and what message you think it sends.

Body Language	What's Happening	Message

… and more to do!

Body language can sometimes be misread. For example, you might think that a boy who is making faces and rolling his eyes at you is making fun of you. But what if his contact lens is giving him trouble? Or you might think that a girl who is rubbing her hands together is cold, or perhaps worried, but it's possible that she just put on hand lotion. So if you're in doubt about the message someone is sending you, you might want to ask what the person means.

Have you ever misunderstood another person's body language? Tell what happened.

_____

_____

_____

Has anybody else ever misunderstood your body language? Tell what happened.

_____

_____

_____

_____

_____

_____

_____

_____

Exercise 33 communicating clearly

---

for you to know

Anger is often a result of miscommunication or misinterpretation. Being sure that you have all the facts before you react, trying to see another's perspective, and discussing your feelings with that person are all important steps in controlling your anger.

Miscommunication occurs when people don't relay their ideas effectively. Here's an example.

Jose told Robert that he was going to the football game Friday night and that his parents could take Robert home after the game. Robert made arrangements with his own parents to drop him off at the game. He told them that he didn't need a ride home because Jose's parents were going to give him a lift.

Friday at the pep rally, Jose called across the bleachers that he couldn't go to the game. Robert didn't really hear him, but waved back. That night Robert went to the game and afterward looked everywhere for Jose. He texted him and left phone messages, but there was no response. Robert finally gave up and called his parents (who were out for the evening) to come and get him.

When Jose called on Saturday, Robert burst out, "Where were you, man? I had to get my parents to come for me, and they were ticked! They had made plans because I told them you'd give me a ride home." Jose answered, "I told you at the pep rally that I couldn't go. You waved back, so I thought everything was cool."

This is a classic case of miscommunication that might not have happened if Jose and Robert had spoken face-to-face.

Misinterpretation occurs when we don't have all the information and try to fill in the gaps—and get it all wrong. Look at the following example of how

misinterpretation can have a negative outcome.

Alexa just couldn't wait to tell Victoria the exciting news: she had just been chosen to represent their school in a statewide competition. When she got to math class, she rushed over to the seat next to Victoria. When Joey came in, he found Alexa in his seat. "She's always trying to get under my skin," he thought. "She knows that's my seat!" He said loudly, "Get out of my seat!"

"In a minute," Alexa answered. "No, now. Move it before I move you," Joey retorted. "Chill out, I said in a minute," Alexa said, and she went back to whispering to Victoria. Meanwhile, Joey was getting angrier. He leaned forward and shoved Alexa — and ended up in the principal's office.

Have you ever misinterpreted a situation only to end up in trouble? Misinterpretation can be a web that traps you. Be careful not to make assumptions about another's behavior. If you get it all wrong, then you're settingyourself up for problems.

for you to do

Tell   about   a   time   when   you   were   caught   in

_____

_____

_____

_____

_____

_____

_____

How could you have unraveled the web in this situation? For example, could you have gotten all the information before reacting? Could you have asked questionswhen you weren't sure of something?

_____

_____

_____

_____

_____

_____

... and more to do

Here's a fun Exercise to help illustrate how miscommunication occurs. You'll need a group of friends to play this game with you (the more people the better). Ask the last person on your list to report back to you so that you can record the final message. You can use text messaging, phones, e-mails, blogs, or any other type of communication. Just make sure your friends know it's a game!

Write down a statement that you're going to pass along.

_____

_____

Record the final statement that made its way back to you.

_____

_____

_____

How did the message change?

_____

_____

How do you think this Exercise applies to real-life situations?

_____

_____

_____

Exercise 34 being assertive

---

for you to know

Assertiveness means standing up for yourself and communicating your feelings without harming others or violating their rights. Being assertive, rather than passive oraggressive, is the best way to get along with other people.

In communicating, some people are passive and some are aggressive, but the ones who are usually liked best are assertive. Let's say you hear that a group ofyour friends are going to the movies on Friday night. You haven't been invited but would like to go. These three reactions can help you see the difference in communication styles: **Passive:** "I'm not doing anything Friday night. Anythinggoing on?"

Aggressive: "I'll be there. What time and where?"

Assertive: "I'd really like to join you. Is that okay?"

Being assertive means

- speaking up for your rights while still respecting the rights of others;calmly and clearly expressing how you feel;

- being confident;

- not letting others impose their feelings and beliefs on you;being able to say no.

for you to do

Read the following situation. Underline Jeremy's inappropriate or aggressive words and actions. Then rewrite the situation so that Jeremy is assertive. Some possibilities include asking to speak to his teacher after class, talking to her before his feelings had become so intense, involving a school counselor, or asking his parents to meet with his teacher. Can you think of others?

Jeremy hated math class. It seemed like no matter what he did, Mrs. Stewart wason his case 24/7. One morning, he raised his hand to answer a question. When Mrs. Stewart looked around the room and called on someone else, Jeremy rolledhis eyes and let out a loud sigh. Later, when he leaned over to talk to a girl in the next row, Mrs. Stewart said, "Jeremy, I'm tired of your interrupting my class. You'll be staying after school for detention." Jeremy slammed his hand on the desk and burst out, "That's so unfair! No matter what I do, you're always on mycase."

_____

_____

_____

_____

_____

_____

_____

_____

... and more to do!

These questions will help you see how assertive you are.

Do you volunteer your ideas even if they are different from others' ideas?	☐ Yes	☐ No
Do you ask questions when you don't understand something?	☐ Yes	☐ No
Do you say no without feeling guilty when you don't want to do something?	☐ Yes	☐ No
Do you speak up when others try to take advantage of you?	☐ Yes	☐ No
Do you face difficult situations rather than avoiding them?	☐ Yes	☐ No
Can you take criticism without getting angry?	☐ Yes	☐ No
Are you able to express your feelings and be receptive to how others feel?	☐ Yes	☐ No

If you answered no to at least three of these questions, you might want to revisitthese earlier activities: Exercise 29 Using I-Messages

Exercise 30 Good Listening Exercise 32 Body Language Exercise 33

Communicating Clearly

Remember, you have the right to express how you feel about things. You have the right to say no. You have the right to speak the truth. You have the right to disagree. You have the right to be you! The more you practice being assertive, the easier it will become.

Exercise 35 steps toward change

---

for you to know

It's likely that throughout your life you will face the need to change. Changing yourself is not easy; it takes time, energy, and motivation. But you can do it!

Your response to anger can change if you

- recognize your anger is a problem;

- explore ways to change your response to anger;

- ractice the skills you've learned.

How long does it take to change your response to anger? Some experts say thatto move from being a very angry person to a moderately angry person takes about ten weeks. So be patient with yourself. It is also important to remember that you may find yourself going back to your old ways of handling anger at times. If that happens, revisit your anger goals and reaffirm your commitment toreaching them.

for you to do

Go back to Exercise 3 and review the anger goals you set for yourself. Write down those goals and the action plans you came up with, and record your progress.

Long-Term Goal:

_____

_____

Action Plan:

1. _____

2. _____

3. _____

What steps have you taken to meet your long-term goal?

_____

_____

_____

If you have not yet reached this goal, what more can you do to help you getthere?

_____

_____

_____

Short-Term Goal:

_____

_____

Action Plan:

1. _____

2. _____

3. _____

What steps have you taken to meet your short-term goal?

_____

_____

_____

If you have not yet reached this goal, what more can you do to help you getthere?

_____

_____

_____

… and more to do!

When I feel myself getting angry, I can

1._____.

2._____.

3._____.

4._____.

5._____.

These people can help me manage my anger:

1._____.

2._____.

3._____.

4._____.

5._____.

I will try my hardest never to_____.

The most important thing I have learned about managing my anger is

_____

_____.

The answers you have just written down are like a snapshot of what you havelearned and how you have changed. Congratulate yourself!

Exercise 36

seeing how far you have come

---

for you to know

When you first started this workbook, you were having a hard time handling your anger. By completing these activities, you have probably learned a number of ways to manage your angry feelings.

At this point, it is likely that you have seen a change in your behavior and that others have noticed as well. What you have learned from doing the activities will not prevent you from ever experiencing anger again, but you will know how to keep it under control. See how far you have come!

for you to do

For each of these statements, circle the answer that best describes you.

I have improved my response to anger.

1	2	3	4	5
strongly disagree	disagree	neutral	agree	strongly agree

I have more control of my anger.

1	2	3	4	5
strongly disagree	disagree	neutral	agree	strongly agree

On average, I get really angry ...

1	2	3	4	5
every day	every few days	once a week	every two weeks	once a month

Read each statement and check either "Yes" or "No."

People have noticed a difference in how I handle situations. ☐ Yes ☐ No

I have learned different ways to cope when I feel frustrated. ☐ Yes ☐ No

I have involved others in helping me when I get angry. ☐ Yes ☐ No

I know I can change how I handle situations that make me angry. ☐ Yes ☐ No

I have not hit anyone since I have been working on my anger. ☐ Yes ☐ No

The higher you rated yourself on the scales, and the more frequently youchecked "Yes," the less anger is a problem for you.

… and more to do!

Look back at Exercise 1 and compare your answers.

What areas have you improved in?

_____

_____

_____

What areas do you think you need more work in?

_____

_____

_____

Exercise 37 anger certificate

Congratulations. You did it! You have accomplished a lot by completing theactivities in this workbook. You've learned

- to understand your anger and how it affects you;what things push your anger buttons;

- how your family may play a role in your response to anger;how your body responds to anger;

- that anger can be a positive force;

- how to chill out and defuse your anger;

- to change the way you think about situations;good communication skills;

- that you can change.

To celebrate all that you've accomplished, photocopy the certificate on the nextpage and fill it out. Post it in a spot where you will see it often!

CERTIFICATE OF COMPLETION

This certificate is proudly presented to

_____

Your Name

for completing the activities in

Anger Management for Kids

Dated this_____ day of_____

Congratulations on all your hard work!

Potty Training in 3 Days

Easy Toilet Training Handbook to Get Your Toddler Diaper Free without Headaches

By

Laura Candice

Table of content:

Introduction:

Potty training is a major milestone for both children *and* parents. It's the first time you get a clear look into *how* your child learns. It's also an opportunity for you to practice patience and trust in a process that is totally unfamiliar. As a clinical psychologist with expertise in child development and positive parenting and a mom of two children, I know how daunting potty training can be—especially for first-time parents who have never done this before! Luckily, it doesn't have to be this way. In fact, potty training can be an incredible opportunity to bond with your child and learn more about each other. Like any other milestone our children will face in life; this is one that can be embraced and celebrated.

It's normal to worry that you'll fail at potty training. You may wonder, *what if this doesn't work? What does that say about me as a parent?* And although diapers smell and are costly, they are much easier to deal with because *you're in control.* Potty training is a journey that requires you to place control in your child's hands. You teach them the skills, provide the structure, and empower and encourage them along the way, but then it's up to them.

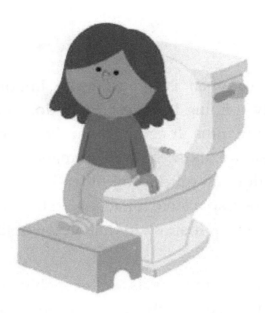

Keep in mind that one size does not fit all in potty training. Every child is unique, and developmental milestones play a huge role in the success (or setbacks) of potty training. Furthermore, children have their own thoughts and opinions. They ultimately call the shots here, but *you* make all the difference in how this process goes. You are their teacher. You provide safety and boundaries, as well as a loving environment in which they will thrive. I'm here to empower you in your role and help you navigate this uncharted territory. You *will* succeed, and your child *will* be potty trained. I will be here every step of the way, with practical and positive suggestions to help make the process more intuitive and fun.

Chapter 1: When to start?

Let state this simply: when is almost more important than how. Unequivocally, potty training is easiest when done between the ages of twenty and thirty months. It certainly can be done earlier or later, with caveats. For instance, most children younger than twenty months won't connect the dots as quickly as older kids do, which means you'll need to be more responsible for acting on their cues (as opposed to expecting them to act on their own) than you would be if they were older.

However, before twenty months is unbelievably easier than after thirty months. Kids over thirty months are that much more sophisticated and skilled at manipulation. They know the power of choice and free will. My mom likes to say, "You want to do it before they know they have a choice in the matter." Anyone with a three-year-old can tell you they are very adept at exerting their will. Your power struggles will be huge. And guess what? You won't win.

Smack-dab in the middle of that twenty- to the thirty-month-age range is best for most people. Right around twenty-four months is ideal. At this age, your child is eager to please, is connecting a lot of the dots in the big world around him, is still malleable, and is dying for more responsibility. Think about it. Kids at this age love helping and feeling important. They want to help cook and clean and do chores around the house — it's the perfect time to hand them their very own responsibility. You want to take advantage of this eager-to-please phase. It's natural, and it's good, and, unfortunately, it will go away. Trust me.

Mind you; there are always going to be exceptions. More recently, I've seen an increase in moms who know their kids are very capable of potty training before twenty months. And of course, there are plenty of children who potty train just fine in the thirty- to thirty-six-month age range. Still, in my experience, this age range is when things start getting tricky.

Why this time frame?

1. There are certain "windows of opportunity" in development, during which a developmental task can be accomplished with the least amount of conscious effort on the part of the child. There are many such windows of opportunity during childhood. For example, weaning. Many kids wean at twelve months because it's usually very easy to do at that particular age. Four months, twelve months, twenty-four months, and thirty months are documented windows of opportunity for easy weaning. Can it be done at other times? Sure, it just requires a little more effort on the part of both mother and child. Similarly, there's a window of opportunity for learning a language. Researchers and parent's alike know-how effortlessly a child picks up a second language before the age of five. The same is true for learning a first language. I once worked with a child who had been secluded in a studio apartment for all of her five years of life with her drug-addicted mother. Because of her limited social exposure, she missed the window of opportunity to learn her first language, English. To this day, she requires major speech therapy and struggles in school. If you want to potty train with the least amount of effort, the window of opportunity is between twenty and thirty months. It's just easier, that's all.

   This period of time is also a developmental window during which there appears to be almost a lull in learning new skills. Your child has probably learned the basics, like eating, walking, and working through separation anxiety. During this period, he is really just honing his skills. Nothing too momentous is being "worked out" developmentally during this time. Note that windows are relative to one another, though, so if your child has had delays in other big milestones, he will naturally be a bit delayed in potty training.

2. Teaching a child to use the potty imparts her with dignity and self-respect. At this age, your child is learning at the speed of light. You're probably amazed and amused by what she is now capable of. Capable of. Do not underestimate what your child is capable of. I see tons of parents gleefully showing off their child's genius while that same kid is sitting in her own poop. That's not right. It's insulting to your child's intelligence to think she can't learn this new skill.

3. For several reasons, if you wait too long after thirty months, the process of potty training becomes a chore for you as well as for your child. There will be fights and power struggles, and things will get ugly fast. It will take too much longer. In my experience, if your child isn't fully trained by four, the likelihood of a child being a bed wetter is increased by 50 percent. You want to try on low self-esteem? Try going to your first sleepover and wetting the bed.

4. Also, as I've mentioned, after thirty months, your child will be well into the process of individualization, that psychological process in which your child learns that he is his own person and that he is separate and distinct from you. This process is marked by defiance and resistance as he learns to express his free will. This process is normal, but things get ugly if you wait until then to potty train.

5. This ideal potty-training time frame is usually accompanied by other markers, which I look for even before I look at age:

   • Does your child retreat to a corner or private place to poop?

   • Can your child recite the "ABC" song?

   • Can your child communicate his needs? By this, I mean:

Can your child somehow ask for water, juice, or milk when he's thirsty?

Can your child somehow ask for a snack when he's hungry?

Can your child throw a tantrum for candy at the market? Can your child throw a tantrum for just about anything?

If your child is retreating to some private place—any place: under the table, another room, maybe even just turning his back—to poop, it is absolutely time to start potty training. Your child is showing embarrassment. To be clear, these bodily functions are normal, and you should not embarrass your child about them. However, with socialization comes a sense of shame in performing bodily functions in front of others. If you were sitting in my class and pooped in your pants, you'd be embarrassed. I'm warning you—if you don't recognize this sign of readiness and act on it, your child will soon forget to be embarrassed. When this happens, you end up with a five-year-old who's not bothered at all by pooping in his pants.

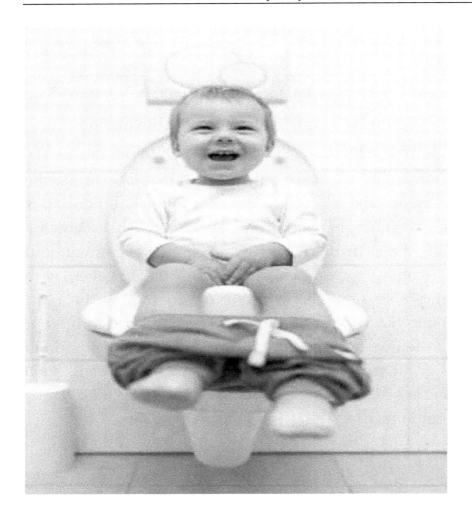

Chapter 2: Mental preparation

This chapter is all about getting your head screwed on tight so it doesn't blow off—aka preparation for the big day!

I know you are chomping at the bit for the actual potty training, but making sure your head is screwed on tight is a very important part of the how-to (actually, it's an important part of parenting, in general).

The very first thing we have to do is to get rid of any notion you might have of how long this process should take. I've already stated my piece about magical three-day training. Yes, it can take a child three days to potty train. It can also take one day. And it can also take seven. I find it very interesting that everyone adores the uniqueness of their children—we love that each one is as different and special as a snowflakee.

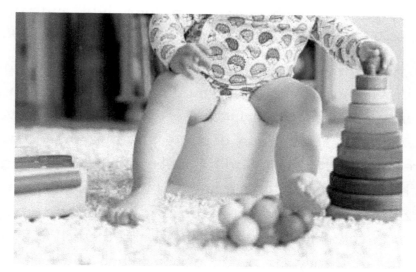

While there is many potty training "methods," there are really only two general systems floating around out there:

1. Rewards

2. Consistency and commitment

That's it.

We are going to work within the second system. Your child is special; she has her very own genetic makeup. She has her very own learning method and speed. We have to honour that, okay? If there were just one way to potty train your child—absolutely guaranteed, no hassles, in three days flat—that crap would be on Oprah (or would've been, anyway). It'd be viral in seconds. We'd all know about it. But we are dealing with humans, who react as individuals and have their own—albeit not exactly logical— thought processes, and who not only know how to push your buttons, they actually installed your buttons.

Using the potty is both one of the first things you actively teach your child and one of the first things he actively learns. What we are going to discover through this process is how your child thinks. Having a preconceived notion of how long this will take is REALLY, HONESTLY going to muck things up for you. You will unwittingly put too much pressure on your child, and you will drive yourself insane. Trust me. I know this.

I see people getting tripped up on this all the time. You want to potty train with consistency, and you don't want it to take a year. Realistically, I can tell you it takes most people around seven to ten days. Through all my years of doing this, I've come to believe that there's a truly magical window of about two weeks' duration in each child's life during which he will potty train so effortlessly it's amazing. However, when those two weeks are going to happen for anyone kid is anyone's guess, and there's no outward signal as to when they are occurring. So, when you hear one of those miraculous stories from your friend/neighbour/sister, they got lucky, is all.

Before you actually begin any potty training, you will need to do a few things in preparation for getting started.

Set a date.

To start the method, you need to choose a date. Any start date may be chosen. Typically, I suggest beginning around two weeks after reading this novel, but really, it's all right tomorrow, too. The waiting time of two weeks is to brace you to have a rest for your mind. Chances are, you've been spending much time recently reading up on potty training, worrying about it, asking across the playground, fending off the understand exactly, and any time you adjust a diaper, feeling a little bad. Do NOT allow yourself 2 weeks to worry about it. Set a date that will encourage you and, ideally, your wife for three or four days to concentrate entirely on potty training. Weekends on holiday are great. When people chose a date to initiate an exercise regimen, a diet, or to stop smoking, this is the same kind of planning time that people go through. This brings you the last hoorah. For those two weeks, fix your date or luxuriate in diapers. The waiting time often trains you for a big change from newborn to the little guy in your child's life. I notice certain parents are scared to give up their babies. It's a bittersweet moment, and it's worth examining for yourself. My own philosophy is that we shouldn't want to keep our kids back in order to meet our own emotional needs. I'll share few suggestions in a little bit to support both you and your child deal with the feelings of the transfer.

Get a potty chair, or if you already have one out, put it in hiding.

The "put the pot out so they could get used to it" error has been created by any single parent that has attended a potty-training class. If it's not put out by you, don't. If you used it to piss and poop in, and your kid has never just used it, you should leave it out. If, except peeing and pooping, the potty chair has been used for something else, throw it away.

I still don't consider making your kid choose a potty chair of her own. Inevitably, they would choose one of bells and whistles, and that's not what you need. It's not a toy here. Personally, I'm a big fan of the potty chairs by Baby Björn. If, between now and your chosen start date, your child wants to use the potty chair, go ahead and let him. So, claim you've set a start date from now on for two weeks. He was using the potty, albeit incoherently. Nonetheless, it's in the toilet and hasn't been some form of toy. You might keep that out. If he asks to use it during the 2 weeks from now until your start date, let him. Don't make a huge deal about it, though. Only mean, "Thank you for using the potty." Potty training is not going to be discussed. You would not offer accolades. Only go back to him with a quick thank you or a reflection: "You used a potty chair to pee inside." Thanks to you.

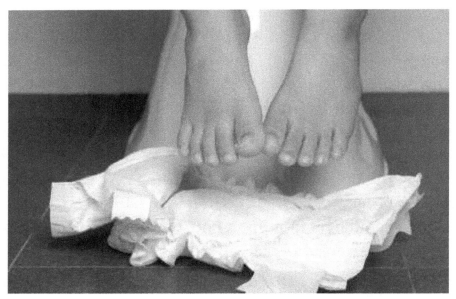

One Week Before the Big Day

Start talking about throwing away diapers. Don't mention potty training. Don't mention anything about the toilet or pee or poop. Just mention as you're changing diapers, "On Sunday, we're going to throw your diapers away." This should be level and calm and very loving. Don't show your nerves, and don't make it a big deal. The logic behind this is it's not wrought with anxiety. Who can't throw away a few diapers? Jeez, Mom. That's easy.

This is also a great time to start with big boy/girl talk. Start going through the list of big kid stuff your child does. Kids love hearing about what they can do now that they couldn't do as a baby. This is preparing both you and your child for the end of this baby's portion of her life.

This particular phase in your child's life is also a place in which your language can generate a mixed message. See if these sounds familiar:

"Who's my baby?"

"No, honey, that's not for little kids."

"Stop that now; you're a big girl."

So, what is your child? A big kid, a little kid, or a baby?

It may not seem like that big a deal, but being able to recognize and address this will come in handy. Sometimes our big kids need babying, and it's good when they can separate and articulate that. One child I worked with years ago came up with the phrase "I need some baby love." I thought this was brilliant and adopted it when training my own son. It worked like magic. Kids aren't so afraid of becoming a "big kid" if they know they can have some "baby love" when they need it. Right now, they're in limbo; we know they aren't really big kids, but they aren't babies either. To this day, Pascal asks for "baby love" (actually, he calls it Mama Love, but it means the same). It lasts about thirty seconds, and then he's on to bigger and better "big boy" things. Still, it gives us that infusion of love and snuggles we both crave.

So, you've set a date, ideally giving yourself a two-week head start. You've put the potty chair away for now. You've cleared your social calendar for a week. And you've planted the idea, super casual-like, that you are tossing diapers out.

Sleep

Yes, we are moms. We are the legions of the underrated. I'm talking about you, but more importantly, I'm talking about your child. Our children as a whole are grossly sleep-deprived. A two-year-old needs around twelve hours of sleep a day and most don't get anywhere near that much. The craziest thing about sleep is that a tired kid acts like a wired kid. So, when it's around seven in the evening, and you think your kid isn't tired because he's chasing the dog around in circles, you're likely wrong. That kid is probably overtired. Another important sign of an overtired kid is if bedtime is a fiasco. Bedtime shouldn't be a hassle. If it is, chances are your child is overtired. Overtired kids are clumsier, have more freak-outs and tantrums, "poke" at others, and are generally fussier. "No, I want the pink cup. No. The blue cup. No. The pink cup." You know the drill. Of course, toddlers are known for their fickleness, but tired kids tend to go above and beyond with regard to the crazy. Fix sleep before beginning potty training. Always, always go for more sleep. If you and your child have been struggling with sleep, please get help before potty training. My go-to sleep expert is Alanna McGinn of The Good Night Sleep Site. She's amazing at getting parents and children back on track with good, healthy sleep habits. I'm not going to spend a whole lot of time talking about sleep, but you really want this duck in the row before you begin.

Potty train the kid you have.

This is a good one. You have the kid you have, not necessarily the kid you want. You cannot change your zebra's stripes. This is hard for us to admit and hard to remember. We all want a well-behaved, loving, courteous child. But we got what we got. And no matter what, our love is fierce. While you are potty training, be careful not to linger in the "I wish he . . ." fantasy world. Deal with the kid and the problems you have. Your fantasies are irrelevant. Wishing your child would be different doesn't serve anyone. There's a lot of "nature" in this here "nurture." The goal is always to work with your child's strengths. While working with a client, I never try to "fix" a perceived weakness.

We build on what your kid inherently has.

There's another aspect to making sure you're potty training "the kid you have." If your child has a particular "problem" before you start potty training—say he's whiny, or she's resistant, or he's prone to histrionics and tantrums—you are going to have that same kid and the same problem while you are potty training. That's not a judgment. All these behaviours are normal, and there's not a single one I have not seen. The behaviour isn't the real issue, in fact. The real problem is when parents somehow convince themselves that potty training is going to happen in a bubble, that all the other behaviour your child typically exhibits is somehow going to disappear while you are potty training. Not only will it still be there—it may even get magnified for a short time. Again, it's all good. Just keep the level of your expectations.

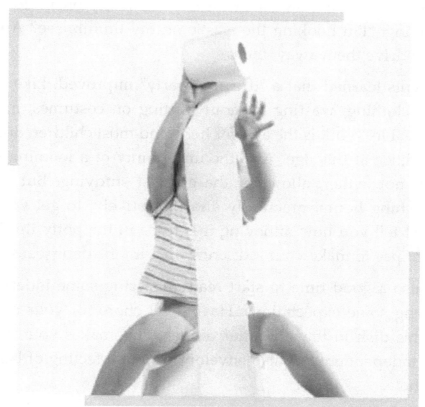

Pants, Clothing, and Independence

Does your child dress herself? You might want to get started teaching this skill if your child doesn't already possess it. I find it's something we don't even really think about until we start potty training, and then it's like

AHHHH!

It will improve a few things. So, first of all, who the heck started to say, "Pull down your pants?" "The Toddlers are too literal. Using the words "Push your pants down" before showing them how to use their pants. That's actually what they're doing, right?

Definitely begin to dress your child yourself. That, in and of itself, is immense. What empowerment it brings them! This often leads to some massive skill-building. It will also take a couple more terms than "I'm putting your pants on" as you instruct your kid to dress herself. Note, this is a whole new talent for her! "So really break down what you're doing: "I'm hooking the elastic on my thumb, see? And I can catch and drive them away, then.

Any parents learned that a "dressing party" improved. Like wearing dress-up clothing, wasting an hour putting on costumes, making it look enjoyable! Work is the answer here, and most children don't get a lot of practice at this age. And the uncertainty of a looming need to pee does not, either, allow for the greatest studying. But set aside some teaching hours, practically and figuratively, to get your pants off. I can't tell you how annoying it is to be in the potty this close to consistent pee to make your kid screw up with the dang jeans!

This is also a good time to start really fostering some independence and setting some expectations. Have a set chore for your child, like putting his dish in the sink after dinner. This makes your child feel big and independent but also envelops him in a feeling of being part of the whole.

They love having and knowing their place in your home.

A Word About Potty Chairs

It's a pretty good idea to have a little potty chair, even if you are morally opposed to them. We really want to foster independence. Your child most likely is a long way away from being able to manage the big toilet alone, even with a step stool. The potty chair is temporary; soon, he will be big enough for the "regular" toilet. I am a fan of both potty chairs and inserts for the big toilet. I have no opinion whatsoever about where you keep the potty chair or how many you have around the house. Buy a pot for every room if you want. I wouldn't worry about any sort of bathroom etiquette at this point. I know some parents feel strongly about only doing poop or pee in the bathroom, but personally, I don't think it matters. Children need the convenience of a close-by potty. Privacy and bathroom etiquette will come naturally with time.

Potty Training a Nursing Toddler

If you are still nursing, right on! That's awesome. The approach to potty training won't be any different, but there is one little twist: because you don't know exactly how much is going in, you have to be a little more alert as to when it comes out. I have to be honest, though: in my observations, breast milk doesn't act like "just" a beverage in the toddler's body. It seems to count as food, as far as the body is concerned. Here's what this means: if your child drinks 10 ounces of water or juice, you can be pretty certain you're going to get at least 6 ounces of pee out at some point. With breast milk, the math is not the same. Do not try to wean your child right before or during potty training! Potty training is a big transition, and your child won't be able emotionally to handle both at the same time. Plus, she may need the stability and comfort of your breast while acclimating to this other big new thing.

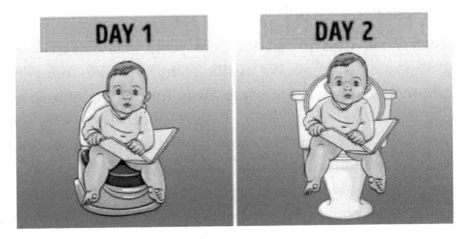

Precious Rugs, Floors, or Furniture

Most people I know with toddlers don't have much that's truly precious. If you do have rooms with expensive oriental rugs or items of furniture that cost more than your house, don't potty train in these rooms. Or make them off-limits for a while. You will freak out when your child pees or poops on these, and there's no greater stall in potty training than a parental freak-out. Casual is the keyword here. Many parents—mostly renters or wooden floor people—confine their child to the kitchen for a day or just until the child gets the basics down.

So those are the major issues you have to tackle to get and keep your head screwed on tight. Once you are clear on those points, believe me. This process is going to go so much more smoothly! Go back and read the chapter again, if you have to. It's worth getting the steps to mental preparation nailed down before proceeding. Once you've got your mind prepared, take a deep breath, and cue up the music from Jaws: dundundundun.

Chapter 3: What to buy for potty training?

Since this is your first-time potty training, you probably need some guidance on getting the right supplies to get started. You'll want to involve your child as much as possible. Remember, young children yearn for a sense of control and autonomy, so you'll want to provide them with lots of opportunities to make decisions during this time. Also, keep in mind that this process should begin weeks before you begin potty training so that you and your child have plenty of time to prepare, both mentally and practically, for the journey ahead. Here are the supplies you'll need.

Chair or Seat?

When it comes to the choice between a potty chair or a potty-training seat, you might have to try out both and see which your child prefers. Here are the pros and cons of each.

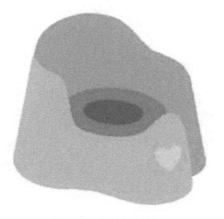

POTTY CHAIR

Potty chairs are often appealing to young children because they sport fun colors, entertaining sounds, and their favourite characters. They are usually much less intimidating for young children due to their small size. They are also easy to sit on and do not leave the child's feet dangling. (Children can have difficulty controlling their voiding muscles when their feet are dangling.) Potty chairs are easy to place around your home for quick access. When shopping for one, make sure to select a chair that is portable and easy to clean. Steer clear of potty chairs that come with splash guards if you have a boy because they can hurt themselves as they sit down.

Where should you put your potty chair? Leave it where your child frequently plays. Ideally, the potty Ideally, the chair will be easy to access to ensure success. Buy a potty chair for each floor of your house will be easy to the downsides of potty chairs are that they can be   access to difficult to clean (particularly poop), and they are often ensuring not available in public places like preschools and success. Restaurants. Furthermore, they can take up space in the bathroom and other parts of your home.

As an alternative, your child can use a potty-training seat that sits on any toilet seat. Your child will be less likely to be afraid of going potty in public if they are used to using a toilet at home. And potty seats involve significantly less clean-up than potty chairs.

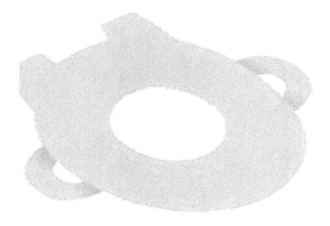

POTTY TRAINING
SEAT

The downside of potty-training seats, however, is that they can be intimidating because of how large they are. Young children may fear they will fall into the toilet. The splash and other sounds can also be a deterrent for little ones. Potty training seats also can't be used in areas without toilets, such as parks.

If you decide to go with a potty-training seat, purchase a step stool so that your child's feet won't dangle. Their feet should rest on a flat surface when they're using the toilet.

Children younger than 30 months generally prefer a potty chair.

Children over 30 months are usually okay with a potty-training seat on an adult toilet. A little trial and error might be necessary as you learn which your child is most comfortable with. Most parents eventually purchase a potty-training seat once their child is older and fully potty trained.

You will also want to purchase a travel potty chair or training seat for when you're in public. There are also travel potties that can be used as a potty chair and a potty-training seat.

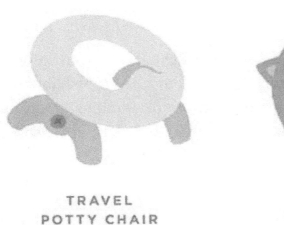

TRAVEL
POTTY CHAIR

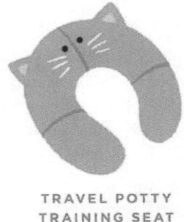

TRAVEL POTTY
TRAINING SEAT

Extra Underwear

While underwear won't come into play until after the first couple of days, you'll want to stock up on lots of extra pairs now. Get your child involved in picking out their underwear by letting them choose their favourite characters and purchasing two to three bags of new, fun underwear. You'll be able to encourage your child to keep their favourite characters dry and comfortable.

Easy-On-and-Off Pants

As your child begins the potty-training process, you'll want to stick with easy-on-and-off pants. Avoid rompers and overalls. You'll also want to steer clear of pants with zippers, buttons, and drawstrings because they're harder for your child to manage. Instead, buy pants and shorts with elastic waists that are simple to remove since your child will be learning the sensation of needing to go and will have lots of close calls. Also, the goal is to teach your child to be as self-sufficient as possible, so clothing that is simple for them to manage is essential.

Rewards

Depending on your personal preference, you may want to purchase small treats, like M&M's, to give your child when they use the potty. Some parents prefer sticker charts or small toys, while others would rather offer simple verbal praise to reward the behaviour.

Flushable Wipes

Stock up on flushable wipes since a fast transition from baby wipes to toilet paper can be uncomfortable for your child. Flushable wipes are much softer than toilet paper and more familiar to your child. However, some children won't mind using toilet paper, so use your discretion on this one.

Cleaning Supplies

Prepare for accidents by having cleaning supplies stocked and ready to go. You will want disinfectant spray, wipes, and paper towels for the inevitable clean-ups.

Step Stool

A small wooden or plastic step stool will help your child get up on the potty-training seat and sit comfortably. It will also give your child a sense of safety and stability while they are high up on the toilet. Your little one will also need a step stool to reach the sink to wash their hands. Some potty chairs convert to a stool to cut down on bathroom clutter.

Exclusive Potty Activities

You'll want to keep a basket near the potty chair or toilet (if you're using a training seat) filled with books, a colouring pad, a magnetic drawing board, and water-reveal colouring books. You can also include toys and trinkets your child might enjoy. Be sure these items are used only for potty time to keep them exciting and fun.

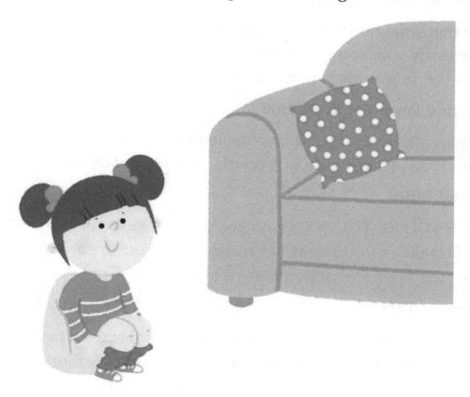

Car Seat and Stroller Protector Pads

Protector pads are a great way to protect your car seat and stroller and relieve some of the stress of going on public outings while still potty training. Bonus: These pads are machine washable!

New Toys and Activities

In addition to the activities to be used during potty time, you may want to buy a few new items for you and your child to do while you remain indoors for the first few days. Play-Doh sets, colouring books, and puzzles can help keep your little one entertained during that time.

Simple and Easy Snacks and Meals

During the first few days, your attention will primarily be on watching your child like a hawk. There will be little time to cook, so stock up on simple and easy snacks and meals for those first few days.

Other theings to Consider

Now that you know the must-haves to get you started, there are a few other items you also might want—as well as tasks to get out of the way—before you begin potty training.

Floor and Furniture Protection

Since accidents are often unavoidable during potty training, you may want to roll up rugs and place towels on sofas and chairs.

Ground Rules

SINCE YOU'RE THE BOSS, you get to set the rules for your child, but as a first-timer, you might not realize that there are a few you must follow too. Here's what you both need to know.

Bathroom Talk (Choose Your Terms)

Before you start potty training, you need to decide what language you are going to use since you'll be teaching this lingo to your child. Your language throughout is critical. It helps your child communicate with you and colors their perception of their bodies and the potty process. Whether you use clinically correct terms like *urine* and *bowel movement* or more informal terms like *poop* and *pee* is up to you. Just stay consistent, and steer clear of words you don't want your child to pick up and terms that carry a negative connotation. It's also ideal if the words are easy for your child to pronounce.

Common words for urination include *pee, pee-pee, wee, wee-wee, tinkle,* and *number one*. Faces is often referred to as *poop, potpie, doo-doo, ka-ka,* and *number two*. There are also several terms for the room where the toilet is located, including *bathroom, restroom, little boy's* (or *little girl's*) *room,* and many more.

For anatomy-related terms, you can teach your son that he has a *penis*. Your daughter can be told that she has a *vagina* and that urine comes out in front of her vagina and in front of where the poop comes out. This understanding will come in handy when she is learning how to wipe from front to back so that she doesn't transfer poop into her vagina.

Find out what terms' caregivers, like day-care staff, babysitters, and family members, use. While it's best if every caregiver uses the same lingo to avoid confusing your child, it's okay if they use different terms — as long as your child is comfortable using those words.

What to Say?

While choosing potty lingo before starting the potty-training process is important, it's also essential to be intentional about the overall language you want to use throughout the journey. Remember, your child is in complete control regarding whether they use the potty. Your role is to empower and appeal to their desire for independence without starting a power struggle or causing feelings of shame or failure. The language you use, and your overall demeanour, will mean the difference between a battle and a partnership.

Here are some recommendations on what to say to make the process easier for both you and your child.

"It's time to go potty."

While your child decides whether they will use the potty, it's up to you to provide the structure. Your child is likely to respond with a simple no if you ask them, "Do you need to go potty?" Instead, set yourself up for success by telling them that it's time to sit on the potty.

"Would you like to go potty in two minutes or five minutes?"

Young children have a healthy need for control and independence. Avoid power struggles by giving your child choices about when they go potty. Pick two choices you are equally fine with (2 minutes or 5 minutes, for example), and then allow them to choose. You can also let your child choose if they want to go on the big potty (the toilet) or the little potty (the potty chair). Giving your child a sense of control over when and where they potty can be extremely empowering.

"We're about to eat dinner. Let's go potty before we eat."

Transitions are your friend when potty training. Teach your child to sit on the potty before and after transitions early on. Prepare them for upcoming transitions by giving them a heads-up about what's happening next and then tell them to sit on the potty first. This is a great way to prevent accidents and create a sense of routine around the process. You can also use *when/then* statements to communicate what you want and what your child can expect after potty time. For instance, "When you sit on the potty, then we can go play at the park!"

"Be sure to go to the potty when you get the potty feeling."

Help your child recognize their body's cues by giving them a simple reminder to sit on the potty when they need to go. Have a discussion with your child about bodily sensations associated with needing to go. For instance, people often pass gas prior to a bowel movement. If you notice this, help your child associate the smell of gas with the need to poop and encourage them to sit on the potty. Recognizing your child's cues (such as the "potty dance") and pointing out the cues at the moment is also a great way to teach your child how to associate bodily sensations with the need to go.

"Be sure to keep your underwear (or character) dry. They like feeling dry and comfortable."

When your child starts to wear underwear, you can encourage them to keep their favourite characters dry and comfortable. This will help empower your child and give them a sense of autonomy and control if they feel they're responsible for taking care of their favourite characters.

"I'm so proud of you for keeping (a character on underwear) dry!"

Shower your child with praise during this process. Be as specific as possible when you compliment your child so that they can learn exactly what behaviours are appropriate and encouraged. Positive reinforcement is a great way to help your child draw the connection between holding their pee for the potty and keeping their body (and underwear) dry.

When praising your child, focus on their effort and hard work (for example, "I see all the hard work you're doing to keep your underwear dry! Fantastic effort!") rather than making vague global statements like, "You're a good kid!" Global statements can lead to a sense of failure when your child has an accident while praising hard work encourages your child to keep trying when there is a setback.

When it comes to praise, don't overdo it or appear too emotionally invested, which can create pressure for your child and take their control away. Instead, praise your child for their successes but keep it short and sweet.

"You're such a big kid. You're going potty just like I do!"

As stated above, young children tend to have a healthy need for independence and control. Praising them for being a "big kid" is a great way to appeal to their desire for greater autonomy. Your child also loves imitating you, so acknowledging the ways in which they are behaving just like you can be extremely encouraging. Keep in mind, however, that this form of praise might not work for every child. Some children become anxious being told they are big kids because they want to continue being treated like a baby. As with any tip in this book, always keep your unique child in mind.

"Let me know when you have to go potty."

As your child becomes more aware of their bodily cues and sensations and begins to initiate potty time, start telling them to let you know when they need to go, especially when out in public. This again empowers your child and encourages greater potty independence.

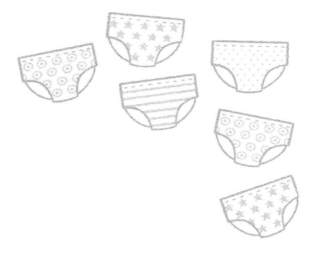

Chapter 4: Step by step training

The first day of the program is probably the most important because it sets the stage for the days to come. Once you are fully prepared, try to walk into Day 1 with confidence and excitement. You got this!

Day-1

Step 1: Have a "Goodbye" Ceremony

On the morning of the first day, you will want to hold a fun ceremony where you (and other caregivers involved) and your child formally say goodbye to diapers. Tell your child first thing in the morning that today is the day they become a big kid once and for all, and say goodbye to diapers. You can say something like, "Today we are saying bye-bye to diapers. You are a big kid now. Pee and poop go in the toilet from now on. Yay! You are going to go to the potty just like me! When you go pee on the potty, you will get a one treat and one sticker to put on your chart. When you poop, you will get two treats and two stickers. Let me know when you get the potty feeling so that I can help you go to the potty."

Start by removing your child's diaper and saying goodbye to that one first. Then go around your home with your child and put all the remaining diapers in a bag or other container. Explain that the diapers will be donated to babies who need them.

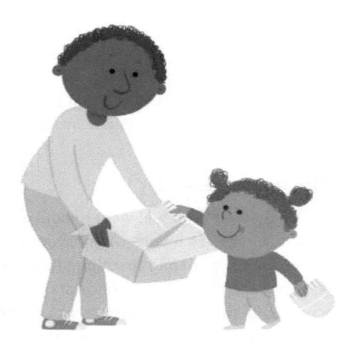

Step 2: Go Naked from the Waist Down

You'll want your child to be naked from the waist down at first. You can dress them in a long shirt or dress. This is important for several reasons.

First, underwear and pull-ups can resemble diapers because they are warm and fitting. This will only confuse your child and increase the likelihood of accidents. Second, being naked is a great way to teach your child how uncomfortable it is to have an accident because they'll have direct feedback on their skin. Third, you'll want your child to be able to get to the potty quickly in the early days. Extra clothes and underwear only interfere with this. Lastly, you're more likely to see exactly when your child is having an accident if they do not have any underwear or clothes on.

Step 3: Orient, Your Child to the Process

After you have the diaper ceremony and remove your child's diaper and pants, let your child know where all the potty chairs (if you're using them) or toilets are and what they need to do if they get the potty feeling. Remind them of what the characters in their potty books did when they got the potty feeling (they sat on the potty). You can even role-play with their doll how to go potty. This all sets the stage for the days and weeks to come, so be as positive and matter-of-fact as possible. Create a partnership from the beginning and focus on uplifting and empowering your child.

Step 4: Load up on Liquids and Salty Snacks

After the diaper ceremony and introduction to potty training, start loading up your child on liquids, watery fruits, and salty snacks. You want them to have as many opportunities to practice going potty as possible, especially while you are in the comfort of your home.

Step 5: Watch Your Child and Stay Close to the Potty

Once your child is loaded up with liquids, it's time to watch them like a hawk. Your child will need your full and undivided attention during this process. During these early days, you'll need to become aware of your child's potty habits and try to anticipate their needs from hour to hour. Catching their accidents in progress is essential. Avoid getting distracted by electronics and try to delegate chores and tasks to other caregivers. Since this can be exhausting, try to get other caregivers involved in the process so you can get an occasional break. Keep the potty chair close by (or stay close to the bathroom if you're using a potty-training seat).

So how do you know if your child needs to go potty? Some common signs are clutching themselves, jumping up and down in place (also known as the pee-pee dance), fidgeting, restlessness, crossing their legs, and passing gas prior to pooping. If they show these signs, calmly say, "It looks like your pee or poop is coming. Let's go sit on the potty." On average, children will urinate anywhere from 3 to 11 times per day, and young children usually need to go to the bathroom within an hour of having a large drink.

Step 6: Prompt and Give Reminders

During the first days of potty training, give your child short prompts and simple reminders to encourage them to sit on the potty. You can say something as simple as "All right, it's time to practice going potty," and calmly and matter-of-factly take them to the potty chair or toilet. Start reminding them every 20 to 30 minutes, and gradually increase the time between prompts after several successful eliminations on the potty with your prompting. The ultimate goal is for your child to respond to the urge to use the potty on their own, without prompts.

Be sure you don't come across as nagging or forceful in your reminders. Avoid saying things like, "Do you have to go potty?" over and over again. Not only is this annoying and frustrating, but the answer will likely be no. Use their cues and the clock to determine when to prompt them, but avoid over prompting to minimize the risk of power struggles.

As they get the hang of it, start to use natural transitions as a way to encourage your child to use the potty. For instance, if you're about to start a new activity, say something like, "I can't wait to play with you! When you go potty, then we can get started." If it's been 45 to 60 minutes since your child's last elimination, or you notice them showing cues, simply take them to the potty and say, "It's time to go potty!" Be fun and light-hearted in your tone, and never force your child to sit on the toilet against their will. Encourage them to sit for a minute or two but don't force them to stay on the potty or to actually go potty before they can get up. If they insist that they don't have to go, accept it and try again later.

HERE ARE SOME HELPFUL PROMPTS AND REMINDERS:

- Let me know when you need to go potty.

- Let me know when you get that potty feeling.

- Be sure to keep dry.
- It's time to go potty.
- When you go potty, then we can have a snack/treat/play/go to the park.
- You're such a big kid going pee on the potty!
- I love how you're using the potty like a big kid.
- Thanks for trying to go potty! I see you don't have to go yet, so let's try again soon.

Step 7: Reward with Simple Praise

Once your child has had a successful elimination in the potty, praise them with a simple, "You went pee in the potty. Yes, pee goes in the potty. Way to go!" To keep your language positive, avoid pointing out where it doesn't go (on the floor or in clothing) and just stick with where it *does* go. Keep this short, simple, and matter-of-fact. While tangible rewards, like a small treat, toy, or sticker, are optional, the American Academy of Paediatrics recommends the use of incentives to encourage your child to learn the necessary potty skills and maintain motivation to keep trying. Just be sure the reward is not so big that it distracts them from the act itself. For instance, one M&M or gummy bear will suffice for a successful urine elimination in the potty. Remember, with any positive reinforcement (whether it's verbal praise or a small reward), be sure to give it immediately after the desired behaviour.

Day 2

Day 2 will not be much different from Day 1 in terms of technique. The biggest new event on Day 2 is one public outing if you and your child are ready.

Step 1: Stay Naked

Your child is still learning how to understand their body cues, and you are still learning about their potty habits. Keep your child naked from the waist down while at home on Day 2.

Step 2: Continue the Liquids and Salty Snacks

Continue to give your child ample amounts of liquids, watery fruits, and salty snacks to give them plenty of opportunities to practice going to the potty.

Step 3: Build Potty Time into the Daily Routine

Now is a great time to begin making potty time a part of your daily routine.

Start teaching your child that everyone goes to the potty throughout the day.

Instead of keeping them on a strict time schedule and reminding them every 30 or so minutes, remind them to go potty prior to transitions. For instance, after they wake up on Day 2, invite them to go potty. After they finish a new activity or ask to go outside, prompt them to go potty first. Of course, if 45 to 60 minutes have passed since your child's last potty attempt, prompt them to use the potty. This is when you want to start phasing out time-based reminders and rely more on your child's body cues and normal daily transitions in determining when to prompt your child to go to the potty.

Step 4: Leave Your Home Commando Style

If you're feeling daring (or going crazy from being inside all day on Day 1) and you think both you and your child are ready, take your child on a brief outing. You'll know you're ready for an outing if, on Day 1 your child had several successful eliminations, and you both are beginning to develop a potty routine. Don't go too far, though! Keep your first outing short (around 15 to 30 minutes); go to a nearby park or run a quick errand. Have your child go commando and wear loose-fitting pants. You can say something like, "Be sure to keep your pants dry. Let me know if you get the potty feeling and need to go potty. I am bringing the travel potty for you to use while we're out." Pick an outing that does not have a time constraint (like an appointment at 10:00 a.m.), so your child uses the potty right before leaving home without rushing. Bring an extra change of clothes in case of accidents. A car seat/stroller cover also comes in handy for accidents while on the go. If your child remains dry throughout the entire outing, give them lots of praise (a treat is optional) and prompt them to go potty when you return home.

IDEAS FOR TRIPS THAT TAKE 5 TO 10 MINUTES:

- Go outside and explore. Look for flowers, bugs, and rocks.
- Watch for clouds or planes passing by.
- Take a trip to the mailbox.
- Walk to the end of the block and back.
- Take the dog for a quick walk. This is a great opportunity for potty talk.

IDEAS FOR TRIPS THAT TAKE 15 TO 30 MINUTES:

- Water play in the backyard.
- Walk a couple of blocks.
- Visit a nearby park.
- Run a quick errand.
- Clean out the car.
- Water plants or the grass.

Day 3:

In terms of technique, Day 3 will not be much different. The biggest change in Day 3 is to introduce underwear.

Step 1: Keep the Liquids and Salty Snacks Coming

Continue to give your child ample liquids, watery fruits, and salty snacks to give them plenty of opportunities to practice going to the potty.

Step 2: Introduce Underwear

If all is going (fairly) well and your child has had several successful eliminations on the potty, it's time to introduce underwear. Throughout the day, praise your child for keeping their underwear (or favourite character) dry and comfortable. This will help them make the connection between holding in their bowel or bladder movements with staying dry and feeling good. This is also a great way to subtly remind them to go to the potty as needed in a nonthreatening way. Keep it fun and light, and say something like, "It's the potty time! Let's keep (favourite character) nice and dry." Keep in mind, however, that underwear can mimic the warm, snug feeling of diapers. If you notice your child having more accidents once you put on underwear, try going back to the commando for a few more days (or weeks) until they have several successful eliminations on the potty.

Step 3: Leave Home

Plan another outing for Day 3. You can make it slightly longer this time (45 to 60 minutes), but don't go too far from home for too long. Just as on Day 2, have your child go to the potty beforehand (but don't rush them). Remind them of the travel potty and the importance of keeping their favourite character dry (if they're wearing underwear), and bring a change of underwear and pants just in case. If they remain dry throughout the entire outing, give them lots of praise and then prompt them to go potty when you return home.

Day 4 and Beyond

The days to come are more of the same. Keep the potty routine consistent. Continue to load up on liquids, watery fruits, and salty snacks until your child consistently has successful eliminations on the potty. Gradually move toward less prompting, and praise your child for keeping their underwear dry and for self-initiating potty time. Follow your child's lead when trying to decide whether to move up a step. For instance, if they are continuing to have accidents throughout the day, it might not be time for a public outing or the introduction of underwear. Just as you were mindful of your child's developmental signs of readiness prior to beginning potty training, you need to be respectful of their ability to handle increased challenges. Move at their pace and adjust according to the feedback you get from them.

The average time it takes to become fully potty trained is anywhere from a few days to several months or longer. There's no hard and fast rule on how long it should take your child to become fully potty trained. Remember, this is not a race, and every child will complete this milestone in their own time.

THINGS TO KEEP IN MIND FOR DAY 4 AND BEYOND:

- Stick with your potty routine.

- Continue to load up on liquids and salty snacks to continue practicing.

- Gradually move toward less and less prompting to promote your child's independence.

- Cut back on rewards once your child has several successes. A sticker chart (if you're using one) is usually the first thing to go. Also, once your child has mastered peeing on the potty, you can begin saving rewards for successful poop trips and/or going a whole day without accidents.

- Expect accidents.

Let's Talk About Poop

Don't be alarmed if your child does not poop in the potty during the first few days of training. Children simply don't get as many chances to practice pooping in the potty as they do urinate. Children also commonly wait until naptime or bedtime to poop or withhold their bowel movements altogether during this time.

The common causes of poop resistance are fear, desire for control, and/or constipation. Oftentimes, children view poop as an extension of themselves and are frightened to feel it and see it in the potty. It can also be scary for small children to hear the new sounds (like the splash of the water after an elimination) and feel the sensations that are involved in the process. To help with this, educate your child on the natural bodily functions of eating and drinking and then eliminating. Read them a baby anatomy book so that they can see how it all works. Also, continue to role-play their doll (or action figure or stuffed animal) going poop in the potty. Use a raisin to demonstrate how the toy pooped in the potty and have a celebration. If you feel comfortable, you can also help normalize this process by showing them your poop and saying bye-bye to it as you flush. Use intentional phrases like "slide-out" and "let it out/let it go" to reinforce the idea that eliminating is an easy and natural thing to do.

Oftentimes, your child's resistance to poop stems from their need to take back control. And as frustrating as this may be, you can't force your child to poop in the potty. Avoid forcing your child to sit on the potty when they don't want to because it can create more fear and resistance. Your child will poop in the potty when they feel comfortable enough to do so. When they poop in their naptime/night-time pull-up (see Chapter 5), try not to get frustrated. Instead, involve your child in the process of putting the poop into the toilet and having them say bye-bye to it. Nonchalantly remind them: "Poop goes in the potty."

The best thing you can do is keep track of your child's poop schedule and encourage them to sit on the potty for around 10 minutes during the times they usually poop. Generally speaking, bowel movements occur 20 to 30 minutes after a meal; simply encourage them to sit on the potty then. Pooping in the potty is a matter of concentration too. Your child needs to be able to sit on the toilet long enough to have a bowel movement. Encourage them to sit for as long as it takes. You can give them an iPad, bubbles to blow, or something else for entertainment to help them stay seated. Keep in mind that pooping is a primal function that oftentimes requires privacy. A diaper offers that sense of privacy your child needs, so if your child appears resistant or anxious to poop in the potty, step away and allow them some privacy.

Also, make sure that your child is not constipated. Common signs of constipation include big, hard, and painful bowel movements, straining during bowel movements, and communicating fear related to using the potty due to pain. You can help alleviate constipation by increasing fluids and fibber in your diet.

Chapter 5: Do's and don'ts for parents

Peeing and Pooping on the Potty in Different Situations, with Prompting or Without

Yay! Block Three is all about leaving the house! Public restrooms can be scary! Always get a good pee before leaving the house. Make it part of the leaving ritual. In the early days, build in enough time, so you have some wiggle room to get that pee before you leave.

- Have Post-its in your purse to cover the automatic flusher.

- Bring the potty chair in the car, so your child has the option to use it in the car if she is freaked out by public restrooms.

- Also, carry a foldable insert with you in a Ziplock for reducing public toilet seats.

- If your child is freaked out upon entering a public restroom, abandon the mission. Offer the car potty chair. Do not push this.

- Always show your child where the restroom is, in both public places and friends' houses.

- At events like parties, be vigilant. Excitement, sugar, and more fluids than usual mean you need to be on high alert. (But don't be that psycho mom, okay?)

- If your child can hold it till, he gets home and there are no accidents, that's awesome. Many adults won't pee or poop outside their own homes, either.

- Bring a spare change of clothes. Keep some extras in the car with some baggies. Accidents can happen to anyone.

- Make peeing upon arrival and/or upon leaving part of your routine.

Peeing and Pooping on the Potty While Naked, Either with

Prompting or Without

By far, the most nerve-wracking days are the first few of potty training. Here are a few reminders in those first days:

- Do not be attached to how long this block takes—usually one to three days but not always.

- Look for progress, not perfection.

- Do not ask if your child has to go; prompt by telling. "Come. It's time to go to the potty."

- Be watchful without stalking. Don't over prompt or hover. This will create pressure on the child and will backfire in resistance.

- Stay off your phone.

- Use easy, natural catch times (upon waking, before and after sitting, eating, car rides, before nap or bedtime).

- This is just another thing you are teaching your child. Lead with confidence, silliness, and creativity.

- Do not post on Facebook. It will undermine your confidence.

- Don't be afraid to use the Red Solo Cup Trick.

- Do not expect self-initiation. If it happens, wonderful. But it won't be consistent, so it's unreliable.

- All you are doing is bringing your child from I'm Clueless to I Peed to I'm Peeing to I Have to Go Pee. Look for progress along that timeline.

- Do not bribe or try to convince your child to use the potty. Blend it in with other tasks;

  "Let's clean up your blocks and go potty and wash hands and then eat lunch."

Peeing and Pooping on the Potty with Underpants On

You are more than welcome to try undies at any point in time. Undies fit snug around the same muscles as diapers and can activate the muscle memory to just pee.

- If the first day of undies brings on a lot of accidents where there were none, it's cool to hold off a bit more.

- Undies are a great natural consequence. If the child wets them, they must go back to the commando as a learning tool, but this can be motivating to the child, so use it.

- Buy a size up, so the undies are not as snug as the diaper was.

- There is nothing wrong with being a commando for a long time. Many adults don't wear undies. If your child does well with commando, that's fine.

- Boxers work really well.

Peeing and Pooping on the Potty, with Clothes On (Commando), with Prompting or Without

Remember that Block Two is the crux of potty training. Most kids do fine naked; it's putting clothes on that changes everything. For some kids, wetting a few pairs of pants is perfectly normal before clicking.

- Use elastic-waist pants for greater independence and because they're faster to remove.

- It's okay to bounce between Blocks One and Two for a day or two. Get a good pee on the potty, and then put some pants on for a while.

- If poop is happening in the pants, go back to Block One.

- Dresses are fine for little girls (and boys, if they like them).

- It's okay to take off pants when you see your child's signal.

- Even if your child begins to self-initiate, you should still prompt. Consistent self-initiating should not be expected.

- If you are being met with resistance, back off. You are most likely hovering or over prompting.

- Use the throwaway prompt; remind your child to remind herself. "Your potty is right over there. Let me know if you need help when you need it."

- Use the phrase "After you go pee, then we can." Don't let this slip into bribery. There's a big difference.

Night/Nap Training (Unless You Are Doing It All Together)

Night training is the most unscientific process ever. Remember that you must usually wake your child at least once in the beginning because ten to twelve hours is a long time to pee.

- Begin the Upside Pyramid of Fluids before actually night training. Once fluids are being monitored, your child very well may start staying dry on their own.

- Night training is possible in a crib. But easier in a bed.

- Two-piece panamas!!! Sleep sacks will make night peeing very hard.

- When possible, leave the little potty by the child's bed. We want to give the child every opportunity to do this on her own if she decides to.

- Don't chase time. If you find you are doing everything possible and there's no discernible pattern, it's okay to rediaper at night for a month or two. While some adjusting of wake-ups may be necessary, don't chase time all over the night. Try to pick up the child's pattern, if possible.

- Night training is never behaviour. The child is never manipulating you with peeing in the night.

Consistent Self-Initiation

Self-initiation is by far the biggest expectation people have in potty training. It is normal and right for your child to need you to help them with potty training. Prompting is a small crutch. Do not remove it too soon.

- Reliable self-initiation usually happens within around three weeks from your start date.

- It can take longer than that. Do not stress out unless your child still needs you to prompt every time after a year.

- Because your child self-initiates once don't mean he always will. Still, be aware of your child's signals, and don't be afraid to prompt when needed.

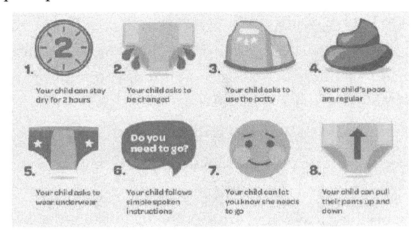

1. Your child can stay dry for 2 hours

2. Your child asks to be changed

3. Your child asks to use the potty

4. Your child's poos are regular

5. Your child asks to wear underwear

6. Your child follows simple spoken instructions

7. Your child can let you know she needs to go

8. Your child can pull their pants up and down

Chapter 6: Tips and dad's cheat sheet

These are things I've found over the years to be tremendously helpful.

Overall, go with what works and be prepared to fend off unwanted advice.

Have stuffed animals, dolls, cars, trains, or any other favourite toy "watch" your child use the potty. This works great the first few weeks. Kids love the idea of showing off to an audience of inanimate objects. It also works great for the child who doesn't want to leave an activity behind. The thrill of the "audience" seems to have limited power, though. Its magic fades after about a month or so (or whenever your kid gets hip to your shenanigans).

Always offer choices. This works well in all areas of parenting. Do you want to use the big pot or the little pot? Do you want to go before Daddy or after Daddy? First, this gives the child some control, which they love. Second, it automatically implies that whatever you're asking them to do is going to happen. But within those boundaries, it gives the child some control. And third, it slips in some learning about the concepts of "before" and "after" and what they mean. Giving a choice works well as a prompt: "Come, it's time to pee — do you want to go first or second?" Giving choices is a great parenting trick in general and can smooth other difficult areas, like getting your child to get dressed. Generally speaking, you should offer two options. Too many become confusing.

Have a "poop book" or two, which are books you keep by the potty or toilet and read-only while pooping. They don't necessarily have to be about poop. There are two reasons for this. First, it helps with the "read every book in the house" problem. Second, it acts as a "prompt" along the lines of a night-time CD. Select only one or two CDs to play at bedtime and only at bedtime, and soon, the music becomes a cue for sleep. In a short amount of time, your child will fall asleep within the first couple of songs. It won't work if you use the same CD to dance around to during the day.] Along those same lines—repetition and consistency—a poop book becomes a cue to poop, and soon your child will poop within the first couple of pages. I'm serious. It's wild how well this works.

An added benefit is that pooping can require some concentration, and introducing new books at a potty time will put your child's focus on the book instead of the poop, while a familiar book will keep the focus where it needs to be. Then, too, you'll probably have the poop book memorized in short order and will be able to recite it for your child when using bathrooms outside your home.

While the book doesn't have to necessarily be about poop, Everybody Poops and anything that combines Elmo with the toilet seem to be kid favourites. Ditto for Elmo on any videos about poop. I personally don't think you need any kiddie-potty videos, but if you can stand them, have it. Elmo = toddler crack. But I'm not telling you anything you don't already know.

Respect privacy. As potty-training progresses, your child will request more and more privacy. Even in the beginning phases, however, while you do have to be present, don't get all up in your child's business. Don't keep looking between her legs or lifting her butt to see if anything is happening. You can be right beside her to assist or read without being focused on the action. Sometimes it even helps to look away or whistle, like you have no idea what's happening.

Make it a habit to show or tell your child where the bathroom is in any new setting, including stores. Something simple, like, "Oh, we're in Target now. You know they have a bathroom over there in the back. Just let me know when you need to use it." When relevant, specify who, if anyone, is available to help. This is great for when you have a play date at someone else's home. Kids get confused—they may know you are a grown-up but may not know that Pascal's mom is also a grown-up who can help. The "status" of teenagers can also be confusing to kids. If you are around teenagers who are willing and able to help your child, you can point them out. This is important because accidents tend to happen more frequently outside of the home due to reduced vigilance on your part and more distractions. Sometimes your time frame for getting to the potty is reduced dramatically when you're not at home.

Be prepared when you're going someplace exciting. Toy stores, carousels, train stations—anything that thrills your child—will most likely bring on pee and possibly poop. Remember: the anus is a sphincter muscle that opens with emotion.

To promote healthy pooping, be sure your child is adequately hydrated. Encourage drinking water over milk or juice. It's better for you and creates a great habit. Be conscious you're not withholding liquids as a way to try to manage accidents.

Be creative and think on your feet. What works today might not tomorrow. Come up with something new. If you come up with a unique solution that works for you, but you've never heard of anyone else doing it, go for it! Every child, and every circumstance, is different. Go with the flow. I remember a former client, Diane, who was having a hard time getting her son Luke to pee in the potty. Luke loved everything about toilet paper. In a moment of insight, when she knew he had to pee, she put a square of toilet paper in the potty. Luke peed in it! That's the kind of thing I'm talking about. A lot of parents get very nervous and want to do everything "by the book," literally. It's okay to use your own creative ideas if they strike. Just about everything is okay if the pee is landing in the potty and you're not doing anything too weird. I'll leave what constitutes "weird" to your own family parameters.

Let it go! I know all this probably seems overwhelming. Don't worry.

It's a lot of information that will become second nature in a short amount of time. You and your child will find your groove. Give your child the gift of responsibility and back off. There's a fine line between watching your child and hovering; learn the difference.

Dad's Cheat Sheet

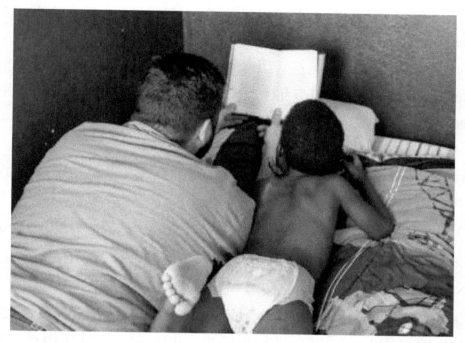

(Once again, I mean no slight to Dads who are reading this and taking part in potty training. I know you're busy, so here's a quick list.)

Hey, dads. So, listen. This potty-training thing has to be done at some point. The earlier, the better. Yes, I know you probably don't want to deal with it when you are tired and come home at the end of the day. And your partner might be a little insane for a few days.

It's all good. This is temporary—all of it. Your kid is going to be so proud of himself when he's done. You will be so proud when he's done. And you won't be spending any more money on diapers. Yay! So please, please, do right by your child and help with this as much as possible.

Here are the major points to remember:

- Your kid is untrustworthy at this point. You cannot just ask him if he has to go. He'll say "no," cause it's his favourite word, and then you are screwed.

- Don't ask, period. Never ask if he has to go. Tell and bring. If you see or know he's got to go —he's dancing around, looking uncomfortable—you say, "Come. Time to pee."

- Use your own leverage as Dad. Your kid loves you in a really special way that is different than how he loves Mom. Use that power for good. Enjoy whatever special time you two have together, but make him pee first.

- Video games, wrestling, TV watching. pee first. Say that. "You pee first, and then we'll."

- Don't act helpless. You know your kid just as well as your partner but in a different way.

- Keep your eyes open looking for your kid's pee-pee dance.

- Don't hover, and don't prompt him every two seconds. Can you imagine anything worse than someone on you like white on rice, asking you to pee when you don't have to?

- Be casual and cool. You probably already have that role anyway. You can be a casual and nonchalant and good cop and still watch out for a pee.

- Your partner is going to go cuckoo. I promise she'll return to normal very soon. Get her drunk. It's okay.

- Do your best to help, even if you don't want to. This has to get done. It might as well be now.

Your role in this is just as vital as Mom's is. Maybe more. Everyone knows that Dad is a little magic.

Conclusion:

Kids may require support to bring themselves to the potty at the appropriate moment, but after a bit, most kids can work out the majority of the potty phase by themselves. These must learn how to wash clean. When kids first come to the hospital for their operations, they are afraid of the nurse and how she touches them and scrubbing them. Parents can first orally clarify why it is necessary to wipe themselves. It is particularly necessary to instruct young girls to keep feces out of the vagina to avoid contamination or discomfort. Girls can clean from front to back as they poop and not from back to front.

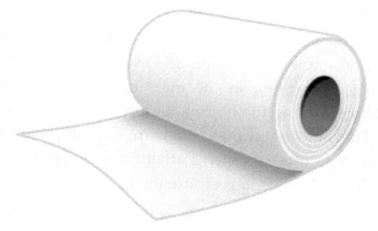

Children can wash themselves after each excretion. The parent can still inquire about the "last wipe" and ensure that the child's bottom is absolutely clean. For more hygienic girls, flushable wet wipes designed particularly for potty-trainees could be a safer option. When small children grow increasingly mobile, and toilet paper is being used properly, parents can educate children on the appropriate lengths of toilet paper for hand washing and prevent excessive finger soiling.

Young children can require assistance with other activities, including toileting. Kids that use self-contained potty seats require an adult to clean and to sanitize each time they use the system. It is a common idea for children to help flush the toilet, particularly if they aren't yet using this. Parents must supervise and guide children's handwashing. While keeping lead safe, parents can often give kids the lead to teach them to keep it clean and germ-free; even that between the fingers and fingernails may also be overlooked.

Eventually, infants understand that they can lose their diapers and are primed for the major moment when they remove their diapers. If this moment also happens, you can still be consistent with leading your kid to the bathroom.

Using a bathroom routine will help children get into the habit of using the adult toilet. Toilets facilitate daily bathroom use, which is nice since it contributes to fewer injuries.

Scheduling a toilet is not complicated. Regularly carry your child to the toilet, for example, every hour, and even when their behaviour is changing (e.g., first thing in the morning, before bath time, after lunch, or before leaving the house). Simply reminding them will not be enough. They may not want to interrupt the enjoyable thing they're interested in to go use the potty. Rather than telling them to use the bathroom, please instead suggest "use the toilet."

And with reminders and enjoyable potty play, new bathroom users would also have accidents. Parents ought to be alert for these circumstances and have a strategy in motion. Be sure to bring little plastic zip-top bags for fast clean-up. Be sure to carry baby wipes or a wet washcloth. Beds should be fitted with water-resistant covers, and at first, infants should also wear plastic training trousers. When injuries arise, parents need to be calm and describe situations to children without getting mad or offended. When Mom cleans up, she will kindly advise Mary, "Your body needed to go pee. Next time, we'll go pee in the potty."

It is absolutely common for accidents to occur during potty training. There are several sources of injuries. Any children will also need to understand how to perceive stimuli until their body wants to remove them. Some children may be overwhelmed since they are preoccupied, exhausted, anxious, nervous, or ill. There are adolescents that have acquired an illness that interferes with bowel function. Children with fever, discomfort during urination, or blood in the urine should be treated by a specialist.

CPSIA information can be obtained
at www.ICGtesting.com
Printed in the USA
BVHW011445110321
602277BV00010B/611

9 781802 240450